Mometrix

TEST PREPARATION

FPGEE®

Secrets Study Guide

AF834552

DEAR FUTURE EXAM SUCCESS STORY

First of all, **THANK YOU** for purchasing Mometrix study materials!

Second, congratulations! You are one of the few determined test-takers who are committed to doing whatever it takes to excel on your exam. **You have come to the right place.** We developed these study materials with one goal in mind: to deliver you the information you need in a format that's concise and easy to use.

In addition to optimizing your guide for the content of the test, we've outlined our recommended steps for breaking down the preparation process into small, attainable goals so you can make sure you stay on track.

We've also analyzed the entire test-taking process, identifying the most common pitfalls and showing how you can overcome them and be ready for any curveball the test throws you.

Standardized testing is one of the biggest obstacles on your road to success, which only increases the importance of doing well in the high-pressure, high-stakes environment of test day. Your results on this test could have a significant impact on your future, and this guide provides the information and practical advice to help you achieve your full potential on test day.

Your success is our success

We would love to hear from you! If you would like to share the story of your exam success or if you have any questions or comments in regard to our products, please contact us at **800-673-8175** or **support@mometrix.com**.

Thanks again for your business and we wish you continued success!

Sincerely,
The Mometrix Test Preparation Team

Need more help? Check out our flashcards at:
http://mometrixflashcards.com/FPGEE

Written and edited by the Mometrix Exam Secrets Test Prep Team
Printed in the United States of America

Table of Contents

Introduction 1
Secret Key #1 – Plan Big, Study Small 2
Secret Key #2 – Make Your Studying Count 3
Secret Key #3 – Practice the Right Way 4
Secret Key #4 – Pace Yourself 6
Secret Key #5 – Have a Plan for Guessing 7
Test-Taking Strategies 10
Foundational Biomedical Sciences 15
Anatomy and Physiology 15
Biomacromolecules 21
Enzymology 24
Cell Chemistry 26
DNA/RNA 30
Microorganisms 31
Pathogenic Microorganisms 34
Microbiology Tests 36
Immunology 37
Pharmaceutical Sciences 42
Pharmaceutical Calculations 42
Medicinal Chemistry 56
Pharmacology and Toxicology 60
Adverse Effects, Side Effects, and Interactions 68
Drug Discovery and Development 71
Toxic Effects 72
Pharmacognosy and Dietary Supplements 74
Pharmaceutics/Biopharmaceutics 77
Pharmacokinetics 86
Pharmacogenomics 90
Extemporaneous Compounding 94
Social/Behavioral/Administrative Sciences 101
Pharmacy Law and Regulatory Affairs 101
Ethical Decision Making 104
Health Care Systems 108
Pharmacoeconomics 111
Population-Based Care, Pharmacoepidemiology, and Public Health 114
Pharmacy Practice Management 117
Professional Communication 121
Biostatistics and Research Methods 125
Social and Behavioral Aspects of Pharmacy Practice 128
Medication Dispensing and Distribution Systems 131

PHARMACY PRACTICE AND CLINICAL SCIENCES — **138**
CLINICAL PATHOPHYSIOLOGY — 138
DATA COLLECTION AND DATA ASSESSMENT — 154
PATIENT SAFETY — 158
DISEASE PREVENTION — 164
PERSONALIZED MEDICINE — 168
EVIDENCE-BASED PRACTICE — 169
FPGEE PRACTICE TEST — **172**
ANSWER KEY AND EXPLANATIONS — **180**
HOW TO OVERCOME TEST ANXIETY — **186**
ONLINE RESOURCES — **192**

Introduction

Thank you for purchasing this resource! You have made the choice to prepare yourself for a test that could have a huge impact on your future, and this guide is designed to help you be fully ready for test day. Obviously, it's important to have a solid understanding of the test material, but you also need to be prepared for the unique environment and stressors of the test, so that you can perform to the best of your abilities.

For this purpose, the first section that appears in this guide is the **Secret Keys**. We've devoted countless hours to meticulously researching what works and what doesn't, and we've boiled down our findings to the five most impactful steps you can take to improve your performance on the test. We start at the beginning with study planning and move through the preparation process, all the way to the testing strategies that will help you get the most out of what you know when you're finally sitting in front of the test.

We recommend that you start preparing for your test as far in advance as possible. However, if you've bought this guide as a last-minute study resource and only have a few days before your test, we recommend that you skip over the first two Secret Keys since they address a long-term study plan.

If you struggle with **test anxiety**, we strongly encourage you to check out our recommendations for how you can overcome it. Test anxiety is a formidable foe, but it can be beaten, and we want to make sure you have the tools you need to defeat it.

Secret Key #1 – Plan Big, Study Small

There's a lot riding on your performance. If you want to ace this test, you're going to need to keep your skills sharp and the material fresh in your mind. You need a plan that lets you review everything you need to know while still fitting in your schedule. We'll break this strategy down into three categories.

Information Organization

Start with the information you already have: the official test outline. From this, you can make a complete list of all the concepts you need to cover before the test. Organize these concepts into groups that can be studied together, and create a list of any related vocabulary you need to learn so you can brush up on any difficult terms. You'll want to keep this vocabulary list handy once you actually start studying since you may need to add to it along the way.

Time Management

Once you have your set of study concepts, decide how to spread them out over the time you have left before the test. Break your study plan into small, clear goals so you have a manageable task for each day and know exactly what you're doing. Then just focus on one small step at a time. When you manage your time this way, you don't need to spend hours at a time studying. Studying a small block of content for a short period each day helps you retain information better and avoid stressing over how much you have left to do. You can relax knowing that you have a plan to cover everything in time. In order for this strategy to be effective though, you have to start studying early and stick to your schedule. Avoid the exhaustion and futility that comes from last-minute cramming!

Study Environment

The environment you study in has a big impact on your learning. Studying in a coffee shop, while probably more enjoyable, is not likely to be as fruitful as studying in a quiet room. It's important to keep distractions to a minimum. You're only planning to study for a short block of time, so make the most of it. Don't pause to check your phone or get up to find a snack. It's also important to **avoid multitasking**. Research has consistently shown that multitasking will make your studying dramatically less effective. Your study area should also be comfortable and well-lit so you don't have the distraction of straining your eyes or sitting on an uncomfortable chair.

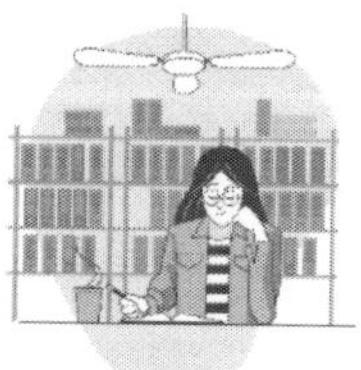

The time of day you study is also important. You want to be rested and alert. Don't wait until just before bedtime. Study when you'll be most likely to comprehend and remember. Even better, if you know what time of day your test will be, set that time aside for study. That way your brain will be used to working on that subject at that specific time and you'll have a better chance of recalling information.

Finally, it can be helpful to team up with others who are studying for the same test. Your actual studying should be done in as isolated an environment as possible, but the work of organizing the information and setting up the study plan can be divided up. In between study sessions, you can discuss with your teammates the concepts that you're all studying and quiz each other on the details. Just be sure that your teammates are as serious about the test as you are. If you find that your study time is being replaced with social time, you might need to find a new team.

Secret Key #2 – Make Your Studying Count

You're devoting a lot of time and effort to preparing for this test, so you want to be absolutely certain it will pay off. This means doing more than just reading the content and hoping you can remember it on test day. It's important to make every minute of study count. There are two main areas you can focus on to make your studying count.

Retention

It doesn't matter how much time you study if you can't remember the material. You need to make sure you are retaining the concepts. To check your retention of the information you're learning, try recalling it at later times with minimal prompting. Try carrying around flashcards and glance at one or two from time to time or ask a friend who's also studying for the test to quiz you.

To enhance your retention, look for ways to put the information into practice so that you can apply it rather than simply recalling it. If you're using the information in practical ways, it will be much easier to remember. Similarly, it helps to solidify a concept in your mind if you're not only reading it to yourself but also explaining it to someone else. Ask a friend to let you teach them about a concept you're a little shaky on (or speak aloud to an imaginary audience if necessary). As you try to summarize, define, give examples, and answer your friend's questions, you'll understand the concepts better and they will stay with you longer. Finally, step back for a big picture view and ask yourself how each piece of information fits with the whole subject. When you link the different concepts together and see them working together as a whole, it's easier to remember the individual components.

Finally, practice showing your work on any multi-step problems, even if you're just studying. Writing out each step you take to solve a problem will help solidify the process in your mind, and you'll be more likely to remember it during the test.

Modality

Modality simply refers to the means or method by which you study. Choosing a study modality that fits your own individual learning style is crucial. No two people learn best in exactly the same way, so it's important to know your strengths and use them to your advantage.

For example, if you learn best by visualization, focus on visualizing a concept in your mind and draw an image or a diagram. Try color-coding your notes, illustrating them, or creating symbols that will trigger your mind to recall a learned concept. If you learn best by hearing or discussing information, find a study partner who learns the same way or read aloud to yourself. Think about how to put the information in your own words. Imagine that you are giving a lecture on the topic and record yourself so you can listen to it later.

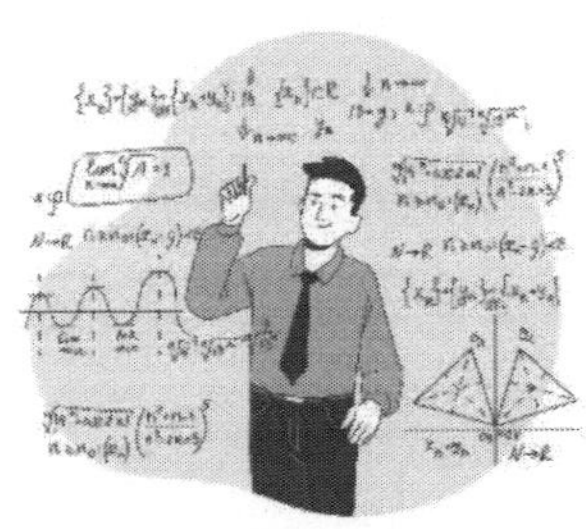

For any learning style, flashcards can be helpful. Organize the information so you can take advantage of spare moments to review. Underline key words or phrases. Use different colors for different categories. Mnemonic devices (such as creating a short list in which every item starts with the same letter) can also help with retention. Find what works best for you and use it to store the information in your mind most effectively and easily.

Secret Key #3 – Practice the Right Way

Your success on test day depends not only on how many hours you put into preparing, but also on whether you prepared the right way. It's good to check along the way to see if your studying is paying off. One of the most effective ways to do this is by taking practice tests to evaluate your progress. Practice tests are useful because they show exactly where you need to improve. Every time you take a practice test, pay special attention to these three groups of questions:

- The questions you got wrong
- The questions you had to guess on, even if you guessed right
- The questions you found difficult or slow to work through

This will show you exactly what your weak areas are, and where you need to devote more study time. Ask yourself why each of these questions gave you trouble. Was it because you didn't understand the material? Was it because you didn't remember the vocabulary? Do you need more repetitions on this type of question to build speed and confidence? Dig into those questions and figure out how you can strengthen your weak areas as you go back to review the material.

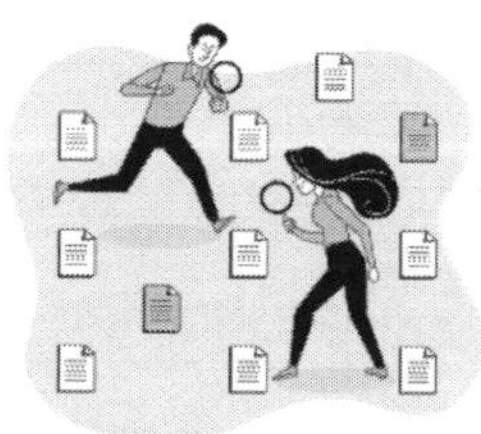

Additionally, many practice tests have a section explaining the answer choices. It can be tempting to read the explanation and think that you now have a good understanding of the concept. However, an explanation likely only covers part of the question's broader context. Even if the explanation makes perfect sense, **go back and investigate** every concept related to the question until you're positive you have a thorough understanding.

As you go along, keep in mind that the practice test is just that: practice. Memorizing these questions and answers will not be very helpful on the actual test because it is unlikely to have any of the same exact questions. If you only know the right answers to the sample questions, you won't be prepared for the real thing. **Study the concepts** until you understand them fully, and then you'll be able to answer any question that shows up on the test.

It's important to wait on the practice tests until you're ready. If you take a test on your first day of study, you may be overwhelmed by the amount of material covered and how much you need to learn. Work up to it gradually.

On test day, you'll need to be prepared for answering questions, managing your time, and using the test-taking strategies you've learned. It's a lot to balance, like a mental marathon that will have a big impact on your future. Like training for a marathon, you'll need to start slowly and work your way up. When test day arrives, you'll be ready.

Start with the strategies you've read in the first two Secret Keys—plan your course and study in the way that works best for you. If you have time, consider using multiple study resources to get different approaches to the same concepts. It can be helpful to see difficult concepts from more than one angle. Then find a good source for practice tests. Many times, the test website will suggest potential study resources or provide sample tests.

Practice Test Strategy

If you're able to find at least three practice tests, we recommend this strategy:

Untimed and Open-Book Practice

Take the first test with no time constraints and with your notes and study guide handy. Take your time and focus on applying the strategies you've learned.

Timed and Open-Book Practice

Take the second practice test open-book as well, but set a timer and practice pacing yourself to finish in time.

Timed and Closed-Book Practice

Take any other practice tests as if it were test day. Set a timer and put away your study materials. Sit at a table or desk in a quiet room, imagine yourself at the testing center, and answer questions as quickly and accurately as possible.

Keep repeating timed and closed-book tests on a regular basis until you run out of practice tests or it's time for the actual test. Your mind will be ready for the schedule and stress of test day, and you'll be able to focus on recalling the material you've learned.

Secret Key #4 – Pace Yourself

Once you're fully prepared for the material on the test, your biggest challenge on test day will be managing your time. Just knowing that the clock is ticking can make you panic even if you have plenty of time left. Work on pacing yourself so you can build confidence against the time constraints of the exam. Pacing is a difficult skill to master, especially in a high-pressure environment, so **practice is vital**.

Set time expectations for your pace based on how much time is available. For example, if a section has 60 questions and the time limit is 30 minutes, you know you have to average 30 seconds or less per question in order to answer them all. Although 30 seconds is the hard limit, set 25 seconds per question as your goal, so you reserve extra time to spend on harder questions. When you budget extra time for the harder questions, you no longer have any reason to stress when those questions take longer to answer.

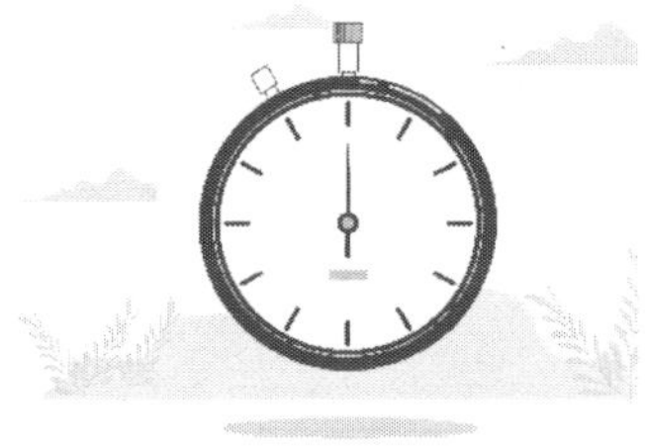

Don't let this time expectation distract you from working through the test at a calm, steady pace, but keep it in mind so you don't spend too much time on any one question. Recognize that taking extra time on one question you don't understand may keep you from answering two that you do understand later in the test. If your time limit for a question is up and you're still not sure of the answer, mark it and move on, and come back to it later if the time and the test format allow. If the testing format doesn't allow you to return to earlier questions, just make an educated guess; then put it out of your mind and move on.

On the easier questions, be careful not to rush. It may seem wise to hurry through them so you have more time for the challenging ones, but it's not worth missing one if you know the concept and just didn't take the time to read the question fully. Work efficiently but make sure you understand the question and have looked at all of the answer choices, since more than one may seem right at first.

Even if you're paying attention to the time, you may find yourself a little behind at some point. You should speed up to get back on track, but do so wisely. Don't panic; just take a few seconds less on each question until you're caught up. Don't guess without thinking, but do look through the answer choices and eliminate any you know are wrong. If you can get down to two choices, it is often worthwhile to guess from those. Once you've chosen an answer, move on and don't dwell on any that you skipped or had to hurry through. If a question was taking too long, chances are it was one of the harder ones, so you weren't as likely to get it right anyway.

On the other hand, if you find yourself getting ahead of schedule, it may be beneficial to slow down a little. The more quickly you work, the more likely you are to make a careless mistake that will affect your score. You've budgeted time for each question, so don't be afraid to spend that time. Practice an efficient but careful pace to get the most out of the time you have.

Secret Key #5 – Have a Plan for Guessing

When you're taking the test, you may find yourself stuck on a question. Some of the answer choices seem better than others, but you don't see the one answer choice that is obviously correct. What do you do?

The scenario described above is very common, yet most test takers have not effectively prepared for it. Developing and practicing a plan for guessing may be one of the single most effective uses of your time as you get ready for the exam.

In developing your plan for guessing, there are three questions to address:

- When should you start the guessing process?
- How should you narrow down the choices?
- Which answer should you choose?

When to Start the Guessing Process

Unless your plan for guessing is to select C every time (which, despite its merits, is not what we recommend), you need to leave yourself enough time to apply your answer elimination strategies. Since you have a limited amount of time for each question, that means that if you're going to give yourself the best shot at guessing correctly, you have to decide quickly whether or not you will guess.

Of course, the best-case scenario is that you don't have to guess at all, so first, see if you can answer the question based on your knowledge of the subject and basic reasoning skills. Focus on the key words in the question and try to jog your memory of related topics. Give yourself a chance to bring the knowledge to mind, but once you realize that you don't have (or you can't access) the knowledge you need to answer the question, it's time to start the guessing process.

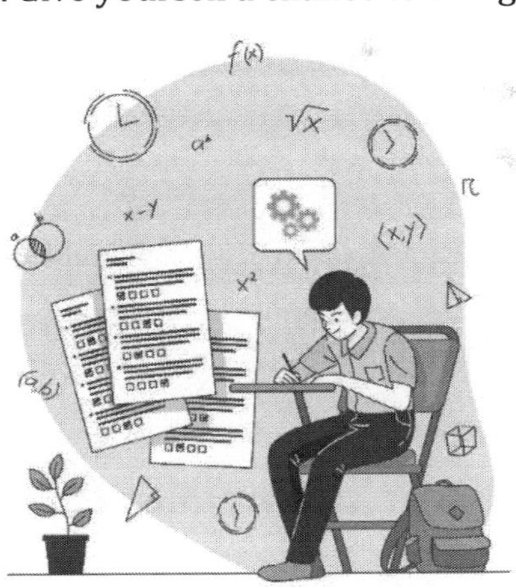

It's almost always better to start the guessing process too early than too late. It only takes a few seconds to remember something and answer the question from knowledge. Carefully eliminating wrong answer choices takes longer. Plus, going through the process of eliminating answer choices can actually help jog your memory.

Summary: Start the guessing process as soon as you decide that you can't answer the question based on your knowledge.

How to Narrow Down the Choices

The next chapter in this book (**Test-Taking Strategies**) includes a wide range of strategies for how to approach questions and how to look for answer choices to eliminate. You will definitely want to read those carefully, practice them, and figure out which ones work best for you. Here though, we're going to address a mindset rather than a particular strategy.

Your odds of guessing an answer correctly depend on how many options you are choosing from.

Number of options left	5	4	3	2	1
Odds of guessing correctly	20%	25%	33%	50%	100%

You can see from this chart just how valuable it is to be able to eliminate incorrect answers and make an educated guess, but there are two things that many test takers do that cause them to miss out on the benefits of guessing:

- Accidentally eliminating the correct answer
- Selecting an answer based on an impression

We'll look at the first one here, and the second one in the next section.

To avoid accidentally eliminating the correct answer, we recommend a thought exercise called **the $5 challenge**. In this challenge, you only eliminate an answer choice from contention if you are willing to bet $5 on it being wrong. Why $5? Five dollars is a small but not insignificant amount of money. It's an amount you could afford to lose but wouldn't want to throw away. And while losing $5 once might not hurt too much, doing it twenty times will set you back $100. In the same way, each small decision you make—eliminating a choice here, guessing on a question there—won't by itself impact your score very much, but when you put them all together, they can make a big difference. By holding each answer choice elimination decision to a higher standard, you can reduce the risk of accidentally eliminating the correct answer.

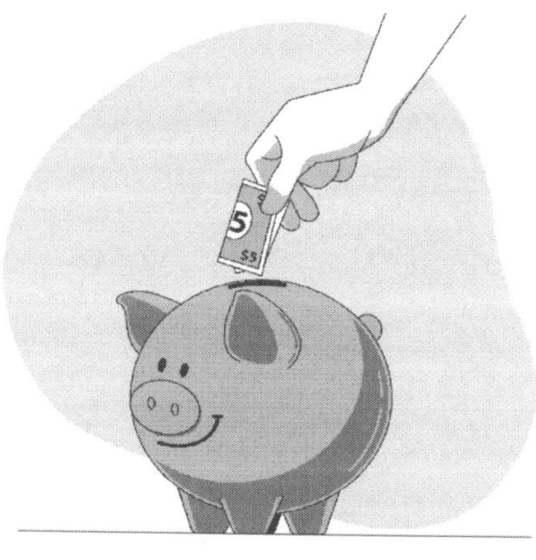

The $5 challenge can also be applied in a positive sense: If you are willing to bet $5 that an answer choice *is* correct, go ahead and mark it as correct.

Summary: Only eliminate an answer choice if you are willing to bet $5 that it is wrong.

Which Answer to Choose

You're taking the test. You've run into a hard question and decided you'll have to guess. You've eliminated all the answer choices you're willing to bet $5 on. Now you have to pick an answer. Why do we even need to talk about this? Why can't you just pick whichever one you feel like when the time comes?

The answer to these questions is that if you don't come into the test with a plan, you'll rely on your impression to select an answer choice, and if you do that, you risk falling into a trap. The test writers know that everyone who takes their test will be guessing on some of the questions, so they intentionally write wrong answer choices to seem plausible. You still have to pick an answer though, and if the wrong answer choices are designed to look right, how can you ever be sure that you're not falling for their trap? The best solution we've found to this dilemma is to take the decision out of your hands entirely. Here is the process we recommend:

Once you've eliminated any choices that you are confident (willing to bet $5) are wrong, select the first remaining choice as your answer.

Whether you choose to select the first remaining choice, the second, or the last, the important thing is that you use some preselected standard. Using this approach guarantees that you will not be enticed into selecting an answer choice that looks right, because you are not basing your decision on how the answer choices look.

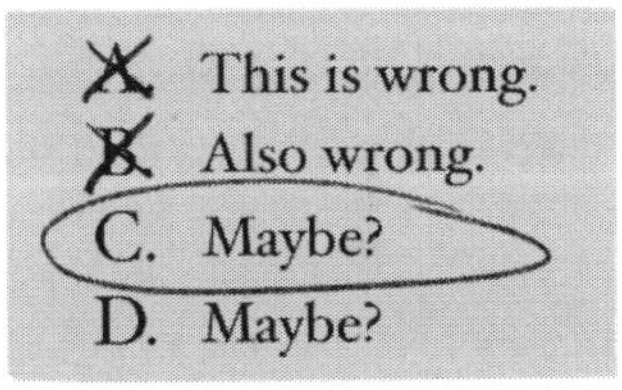

This is not meant to make you question your knowledge. Instead, it is to help you recognize the difference between your knowledge and your impressions. There's a huge difference between thinking an answer is right because of what you know, and thinking an answer is right because it looks or sounds like it should be right.

Summary: To ensure that your selection is appropriately random, make a predetermined selection from among all answer choices you have not eliminated.

Test-Taking Strategies

This section contains a list of test-taking strategies that you may find helpful as you work through the test. By taking what you know and applying logical thought, you can maximize your chances of answering any question correctly!

It is very important to realize that every question is different and every person is different: no single strategy will work on every question, and no single strategy will work for every person. That's why we've included all of them here, so you can try them out and determine which ones work best for different types of questions and which ones work best for you.

Question Strategies

☑ Read Carefully

Read the question and the answer choices carefully. Don't miss the question because you misread the terms. You have plenty of time to read each question thoroughly and make sure you understand what is being asked. Yet a happy medium must be attained, so don't waste too much time. You must read carefully and efficiently.

☑ Contextual Clues

Look for contextual clues. If the question includes a word you are not familiar with, look at the immediate context for some indication of what the word might mean. Contextual clues can often give you all the information you need to decipher the meaning of an unfamiliar word. Even if you can't determine the meaning, you may be able to narrow down the possibilities enough to make a solid guess at the answer to the question.

☑ Prefixes

If you're having trouble with a word in the question or answer choices, try dissecting it. Take advantage of every clue that the word might include. Prefixes can be a huge help. Usually, they allow you to determine a basic meaning. *Pre-* means before, *post-* means after, *pro-* is positive, *de-* is negative. From prefixes, you can get an idea of the general meaning of the word and try to put it into context.

☑ Hedge Words

Watch out for critical hedge words, such as *likely, may, can, often, almost, mostly, usually, generally, rarely*, and *sometimes*. Question writers insert these hedge phrases to cover every possibility. Often an answer choice will be wrong simply because it leaves no room for exception. Be on guard for answer choices that have definitive words such as *exactly* and *always*.

☑ Switchback Words

Stay alert for *switchbacks*. These are the words and phrases frequently used to alert you to shifts in thought. The most common switchback words are *but, although*, and *however*. Others include *nevertheless, on the other hand, even though, while, in spite of, despite*, and *regardless of*. Switchback words are important to catch because they can change the direction of the question or an answer choice.

⊘ Face Value

When in doubt, use common sense. Accept the situation in the problem at face value. Don't read too much into it. These problems will not require you to make wild assumptions. If you have to go beyond creativity and warp time or space in order to have an answer choice fit the question, then you should move on and consider the other answer choices. These are normal problems rooted in reality. The applicable relationship or explanation may not be readily apparent, but it is there for you to figure out. Use your common sense to interpret anything that isn't clear.

Answer Choice Strategies

⊘ Answer Selection

The most thorough way to pick an answer choice is to identify and eliminate wrong answers until only one is left, then confirm it is the correct answer. Sometimes an answer choice may immediately seem right, but be careful. The test writers will usually put more than one reasonable answer choice on each question, so take a second to read all of them and make sure that the other choices are not equally obvious. As long as you have time left, it is better to read every answer choice than to pick the first one that looks right without checking the others.

⊘ Answer Choice Families

An answer choice family consists of two (in rare cases, three) answer choices that are very similar in construction and cannot all be true at the same time. If you see two answer choices that are direct opposites or parallels, one of them is usually the correct answer. For instance, if one answer choice says that quantity *x* increases and another either says that quantity *x* decreases (opposite) or says that quantity *y* increases (parallel), then those answer choices would fall into the same family. An answer choice that doesn't match the construction of the answer choice family is more likely to be incorrect. Most questions will not have answer choice families, but when they do appear, you should be prepared to recognize them.

⊘ Eliminate Answers

Eliminate answer choices as soon as you realize they are wrong, but make sure you consider all possibilities. If you are eliminating answer choices and realize that the last one you are left with is also wrong, don't panic. Start over and consider each choice again. There may be something you missed the first time that you will realize on the second pass.

⊘ Avoid Fact Traps

Don't be distracted by an answer choice that is factually true but doesn't answer the question. You are looking for the choice that answers the question. Stay focused on what the question is asking for so you don't accidentally pick an answer that is true but incorrect. Always go back to the question and make sure the answer choice you've selected actually answers the question and is not merely a true statement.

⊘ Extreme Statements

In general, you should avoid answers that put forth extreme actions as standard practice or proclaim controversial ideas as established fact. An answer choice that states the "process should be used in certain situations, if..." is much more likely to be correct than one that states the "process should be discontinued completely." The first is a calm rational statement and doesn't even make a definitive, uncompromising stance, using a hedge word *if* to provide wiggle room, whereas the second choice is far more extreme.

⊘ Benchmark

As you read through the answer choices and you come across one that seems to answer the question well, mentally select that answer choice. This is not your final answer, but it's the one that will help you evaluate the other answer choices. The one that you selected is your benchmark or standard for judging each of the other answer choices. Every other answer choice must be compared to your benchmark. That choice is correct until proven otherwise by another answer choice beating it. If you find a better answer, then that one becomes your new benchmark. Once you've decided that no other choice answers the question as well as your benchmark, you have your final answer.

⊘ Predict the Answer

Before you even start looking at the answer choices, it is often best to try to predict the answer. When you come up with the answer on your own, it is easier to avoid distractions and traps because you will know exactly what to look for. The right answer choice is unlikely to be word-for-word what you came up with, but it should be a close match. Even if you are confident that you have the right answer, you should still take the time to read each option before moving on.

General Strategies

⊘ Tough Questions

If you are stumped on a problem or it appears too hard or too difficult, don't waste time. Move on! Remember though, if you can quickly check for obviously incorrect answer choices, your chances of guessing correctly are greatly improved. Before you completely give up, at least try to knock out a couple of possible answers. Eliminate what you can and then guess at the remaining answer choices before moving on.

⊘ Check Your Work

Since you will probably not know every term listed and the answer to every question, it is important that you get credit for the ones that you do know. Don't miss any questions through careless mistakes. If at all possible, try to take a second to look back over your answer selection and make sure you've selected the correct answer choice and haven't made a costly careless mistake (such as marking an answer choice that you didn't mean to mark). This quick double check should more than pay for itself in caught mistakes for the time it costs.

⊘ Pace Yourself

It's easy to be overwhelmed when you're looking at a page full of questions; your mind is confused and full of random thoughts, and the clock is ticking down faster than you would like. Calm down and maintain the pace that you have set for yourself. Especially as you get down to the last few minutes of the test, don't let the small numbers on the clock make you panic. As long as you are on track by monitoring your pace, you are guaranteed to have time for each question.

⊘ Don't Rush

It is very easy to make errors when you are in a hurry. Maintaining a fast pace in answering questions is pointless if it makes you miss questions that you would have gotten right otherwise. Test writers like to include distracting information and wrong answers that seem right. Taking a little extra time to avoid careless mistakes can make all the difference in your test score. Find a pace that allows you to be confident in the answers that you select.

✓ KEEP MOVING

Panicking will not help you pass the test, so do your best to stay calm and keep moving. Taking deep breaths and going through the answer elimination steps you practiced can help to break through a stress barrier and keep your pace.

Final Notes

The combination of a solid foundation of content knowledge and the confidence that comes from practicing your plan for applying that knowledge is the key to maximizing your performance on test day. As your foundation of content knowledge is built up and strengthened, you'll find that the strategies included in this chapter become more and more effective in helping you quickly sift through the distractions and traps of the test to isolate the correct answer.

Now that you're preparing to move forward into the test content chapters of this book, be sure to keep your goal in mind. As you read, think about how you will be able to apply this information on the test. If you've already seen sample questions for the test and you have an idea of the question format and style, try to come up with questions of your own that you can answer based on what you're reading. This will give you valuable practice applying your knowledge in the same ways you can expect to on test day.

Good luck and good studying!

Foundational Biomedical Sciences

Anatomy and Physiology

Conduction System of the Heart

Conduction of the heart begins at the SA node. Pacemaker cells in the SA node depolarize. This triggers depolarization of cardiac cells along the internodal pathway between the SA node and the AV node. While this signal spreads across the AV node, the atria contracts. The signal then travels down through the ventricle to the bundle of His, down the left and right bundle branches and then across the Purkinje fibers. This signal causes all the cells in the ventricle to contract at the exact same time causing one uniform contraction of the ventricle.

PQRST on an Electrocardiogram

PQRST:

- **P**: Depolarization of the atria.
- **QRS**: Depolarization of the ventricles.
- **T:** Repolarization of the ventricles.

Repolarization of the atria cannot be seen on an electrocardiogram.

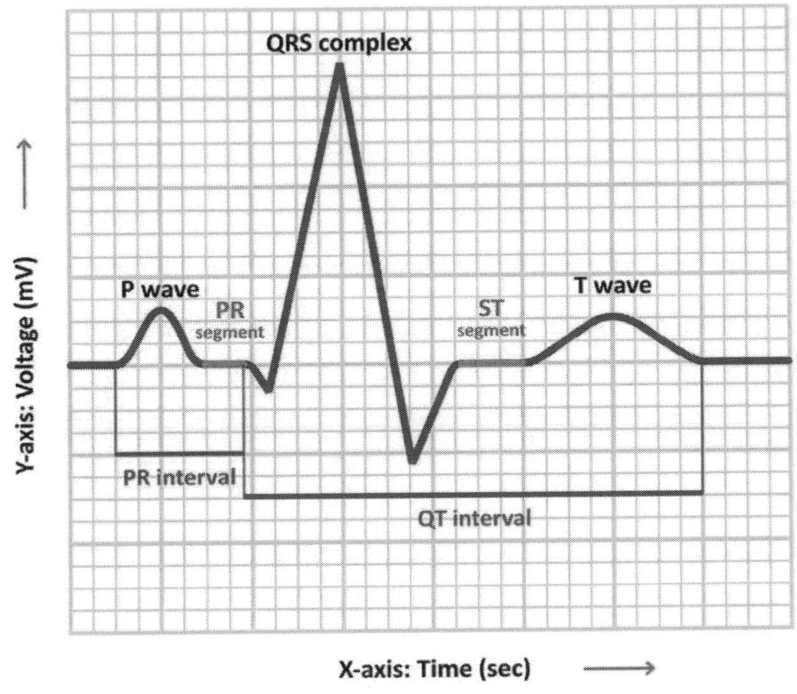

Nervous System

The nervous system is separated into two major components: the central nervous system (CNS) and the peripheral nervous system (PNS). The CNS contains the brain and the spinal cord and the PNS contains the nerves that run signals to and from the rest of your body. The PNS is then separated into two major components: the somatic nerve system and the autonomic nerve system. Somatic nerves are located in skeletal muscle and can be voluntarily controlled. Autonomic nerves are located in smooth muscle, cardiac muscle and most glands and as the name suggests are controlled solely by signals from the CNS. The PNS is then further divided into parasympathetic nerves and sympathetic nerves. All organs in the body are supplied with both parasympathetic and sympathetic nerves. The sympathetic system is activated during activities the body considers stressful (fight or flight response) and the parasympathetic system is activated during times of rest.

Review Video: What is the Function of the Nervous System
Visit mometrix.com/academy and enter code: 708428

Action Potential

Every signal that a nerve sends is done so via an **action potential**. Action potentials occur when a nerve cell membrane reaches what is called the critical threshold level. This is usually -65mV, but can vary depending on the location of the nerve cell. The entire process of producing an action potential is centered on the opening and closing of sodium channels. The initial rapid depolarization of the membrane is caused by sodium channels opening and subsequent rapid repolarization of the membrane is caused by sodium channels closing. Action potentials are propagated via a domino effect. One nerve cell producing an action potential will cause the adjacent nerve cell to depolarize and produce an action potential. The speed of the propagation of action potentials is directly related to whether a nerve fiber is myelinated. Myelinated nerves propagate action potentials faster than unmyelinated nerves. Multiple sclerosis is an example of a disease that damages the myelin sheath and causes muscle dysfunction due to poor propagation of action potentials.

Intracellular and Extracellular Fluid Compartments

At least 70 percent of the total body weight of a person is water. The water content in a human can be divided into 2 major compartments: intracellular fluid and extracellular fluid. **Intracellular fluid** contains higher concentrations of amino acids, magnesium ions and potassium ions compared to interstitial fluid. **Extracellular fluid** is located outside the cell and is primarily composed of interstitial fluid and blood plasma. **Interstitial fluid** contains higher concentrations of glucose, sodium ions and calcium ions compared to intracellular fluid. Cerebrospinal fluid, intraocular fluid and synovial fluid are all also considered extracellular fluid.

Erythrocytes

Erythrocytes (red blood cells) are created in the bone marrow, have a lifespan of approximately 120 days and are destroyed by the spleen. Erythrocytes contain a molecule known as hemoglobin, a molecule that contains heme groups, which allow through the presence of an iron atom to bind oxygen and carbon dioxide. The function of the erythrocytes is to transport oxygen from the lungs to the rest of the body, as well as transport carbon dioxide away from the tissues, to be eventually exhaled from the lungs. Erythrocytes possess important inherited glycoproteins or antigens on the cell surface, which gives an individual the blood type A, B, AB, or O.

Lymphatic System

The lymphatic system is composed of a collection of vessels that are located across the entire body. This system acts to move fluid and protein that has leaked out of capillaries back into the cardiovascular system. This is accomplished by a series of vessels that start as small networks called lymph capillaries. These lymph capillaries drain into slightly larger lymph collecting vessels that are attached to lymph nodes. Lymph nodes act like a filter to help clean the lymph of bacteria. After the lymph fluid has been filtered through the lymph nodes, it flows through the lymph trunks and into the lymph ducts. Lymph ducts drain into the venous cardiovascular system near the right and left jugular veins. When any part of the lymphatic system is damaged or removed, fluid and proteins that have leaked out of capillaries have no way to be returned to the circulatory system and tend to collect in the surrounding tissue. This collection of excess fluid is called edema.

Pituitary Gland

The pituitary gland consists of two lobes; anterior and posterior and is connected to the hypothalamus at the base of the brain.

Hormones Secreted from Anterior Lobe

The following **hormones** are secreted from **anterior lobe** of the pituitary gland:

- Somatotropin (Human Growth Hormone, HGH) — regulates metabolism of proteins, carbohydrates, and lipids. Regulates organism growth.
- Prolactin (LH)—promotes breast milk lactation as well as breast development.
- Thyroid Stimulating Hormone (TSH)—regulates thyroid gland hormone secretions.
- Adrenocorticotrophin Hormone (ACTH)—regulates adrenal gland hormone secretions.
- Follicle Stimulating Hormone (FSH)—important in the regulation of spermatogenesis and follicle development.
- Luteinizing Hormone (LH also known as Interstitial Cell Stimulating Hormone or ICSH)—stimulates development of corpora lutea (lining of the uterus) and ovulation in women. In males, stimulates androgen secretion in males and is important in testes development.
- Melanocyte Stimulating Hormone (MSH)—regulates skin pigment and melanin levels.

Hormones Secreted from Posterior Lobe

The following **hormones** are secreted from **posterior lobe** of the pituitary gland:

- Antidiuretic Hormone (ADH, Vasopressin) — regulates and increases water reabsorption in the kidney during times of dehydration, leading to the excretion of concentrated urine. Also regulates blood pressure.
- Oxytocin—Important during childbirth, stimulates uterus contractions and milk secretion.

Thyroid and Parathyroid Glands

The **thyroid gland** is located near the pharynx. It is an area that serves as a passage for food and air from the mouth and/or nose to the esophagus or the larynx. The **parathyroid gland** is found on the posterior side of the thyroid gland.

The hormones secreted from **thyroid gland** are as follows:

- **Thyroxine** regulates metabolism by increasing the activity and number of mitochondria, leading to increased protein synthesis and breakdown. Essential for proper growth and development of the body.
- **Calcitonin** regulates calcium levels in the blood, and decreases calcium loss from the skeletal bones.

The hormones secreted from **parathyroid gland** are as follows:

- **Parathyroid hormone** regulates calcium and phosphorous levels in the body

Thymus and Pineal Glands

The **thymus gland** is located in the chest cavity just behind the sternum. The thymus gland secretes thymosin. Thymosin is a hormone that plays an important role in the immune system through regulation of T-cell function and maturation. The **pineal gland** is located in the center of the brain.

The pineal gland regulates the day-night cycle by regulating melatonin levels. More needs to be studied.

SKELETAL MUSCLE

Skeletal muscle is essentially long cords of rope-like tissue. Muscle is composed of many muscle fibers. Each muscle fiber contains many myofibrils and each myofibril contains many filaments. Each muscle filament contains thick filaments called myosin and thin filaments called actin. Myosin and actin alternate and are connected by cross bridges. This grouping of actin, myosin and cross bridges is called a sarcomere and each sarcomere is connected to the adjacent sarcomere via a z disc. **Calcium** is the major ion that is required to begin a muscle contraction. Calcium causes actin and myosin to bond together. This bonding causes the myosin head to move in what is called a power stroke. A power stroke essentially causes the actin and myosin filaments to pull closer to each other and causes the muscle to contract. **ATP** is utilized as an energy source for muscle contraction. In this case, ATP is converted to ADP by an enzymatic process in the myosin heads.

CONNECTIVE TISSUE

Connective tissue is derived from an embryonic tissue called mesenchyme. Connective tissue is divided into two types: loose connective tissue and dense connective tissue:

- **Loose connective tissue** contains both adipose tissue and areolar tissue. Areolar tissue can be found throughout the body and is found directly under epithelia tissue. It also encases all nerves and all blood capillaries. Areolar tissue functions as a barrier from infection, a vessel to move body fluids and it helps reinforce other tissues. Adipose tissue is composed primarily of large fat storing adipose cells. Adipose tissue functions as the main storage area for fat in the body. It is located right below the hypodermis and makes up about 20% of the body weight of a normal person.
- **Dense connective tissue** is the main component of ligaments and tendons. This type of tissue functions to help resist tensile forces that joints encounter on a daily basis. Dense connective tissue has a large amount of collagen, which adds strength and allows it to resist tension from a variety of directions.

KIDNEYS AND NEPHRONS

From a basic point of view, the **kidney** is simply an artery bringing blood into the nephrons of the kidney, a ureter to send urine to the bladder and a vein to send filtered blood back into circulation. The main body of the kidney is made up of millions of tiny units called nephrons. Arterial blood flows into the nephron via the afferent arteriole. From there, blood flows through the glomerulus where it is filtered across the glomerular membrane and now called glomerular filtrate. Glomerular filtrate then travels through Bowman's capsule, down the proximal tubule, along the loop of Henle and up the distal tubule. As glomerular filtrate travels along this path, substances that are unwanted are pulled out of the glomerular filtrate and move down the collecting duct and finally excreted in urine. Common substances that are filtered out of blood include: metabolic wastes such as urea, uric acid, creatinine, hydrogen ions, potassium, sodium and chloride.

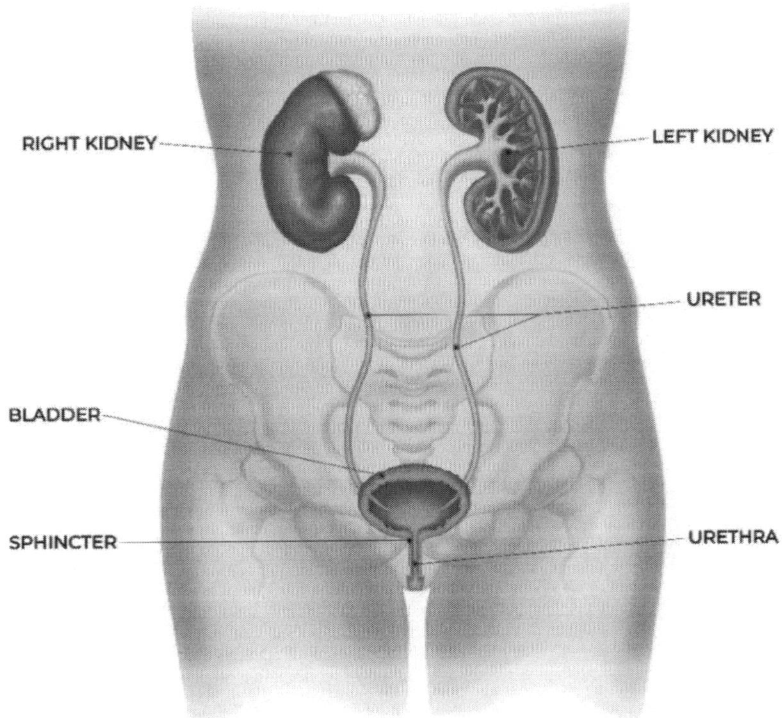

Concentration of Various Substances in the Urine

Substances that can be found in **urine** include: glucose, urea, inulin and para-aminohippuric acid (PAH). Under normal circumstances, glucose should always be reabsorbed by the proximal tubule and therefore the concentration of glucose in the urine should be zero. If glucose is found in the urine, it can be an indication of diabetes mellitus. Only about 50 percent of urea is reabsorbed as it passes through the kidney. Urea is 65 times more concentrated in the urine compared to plasma concentrations of urea. Inulin concentrations in urine can vary, but in general, inulin is 125 times more concentrated in urine compared to plasma concentrations of inulin. PAH is different in that it is a molecule that is both passively filtered into the urine and actively secreted into the urine via the proximal tubule. Urine concentration reflects both passive filtration and active secretion and is in general at least 500 times more concentrated in urine compared to plasma concentrations of PAH.

Gas Exchange in the Lung

In the **lung**, gas exchange takes place along the pulmonary membrane and occurs via passive diffusion. The pulmonary membrane surrounds the small alveolar sacs that are in the lungs. Surrounding each pulmonary membrane is a small layer of capillary blood vessels. These vessels serve as the location where venous blood becomes oxygenated again. As venous blood passes into the capillary bed, red blood cells are oxygenated via oxygen that diffuses across the pulmonary membrane from the alveolus. At the same time, carbon dioxide diffuses from the blood in the alveolus where it is exhaled in the breathing process. Once oxygen has been restored to the blood, it passes through the pulmonary capillaries and travels out to the body via attached arteries.

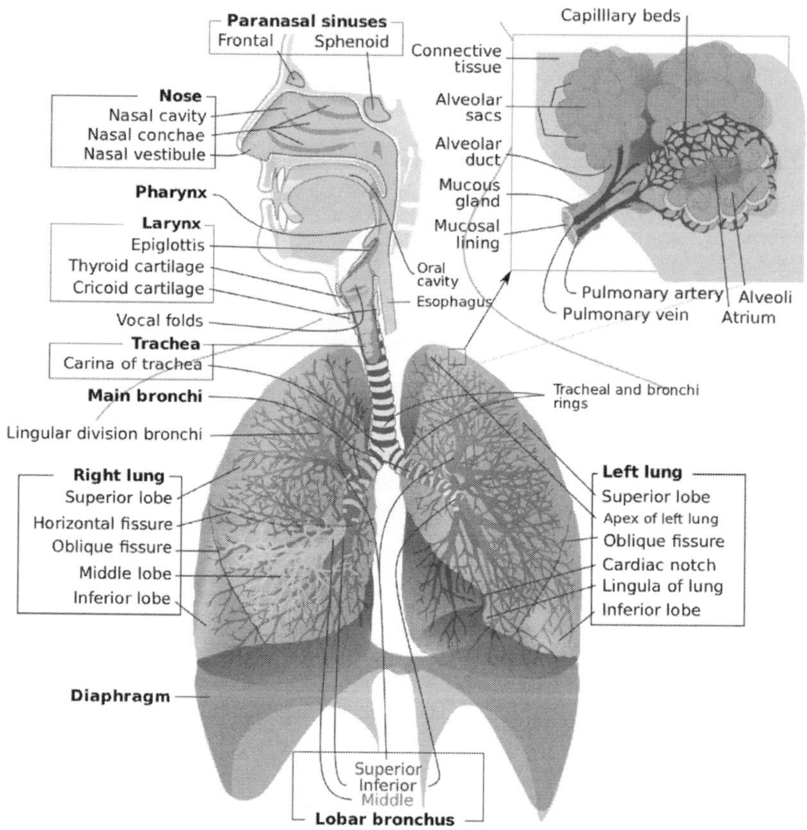

Gastrointestinal Tract

The gastrointestinal tract is a large (over 11 feet) lumen that begins at the mouth and ends at the anus. The gastrointestinal tract is essentially considered open to the outside world and functions to allow nutrients to come into the body and at the same time protect the body from potentially harmful pathogens. This is achieved by cells in the gastrointestinal wall only allowing specific nutrients to pass through the wall and into the blood stream. The gastrointestinal tract begins with the mouth and continues down the esophagus, through the lower esophageal sphincter and into the stomach. In the stomach, food is mixed with acidic digestive juices and mixed via muscle contractions. This mixture, now called chyme, is pressed through the pyloric sphincter and into the small intestine, the major site of nutrient absorption. Chyme then passes through the ileocecal valve and into the large intestine where more nutrient absorption occurs and unabsorbed matter is turned into feces and excreted through the anus.

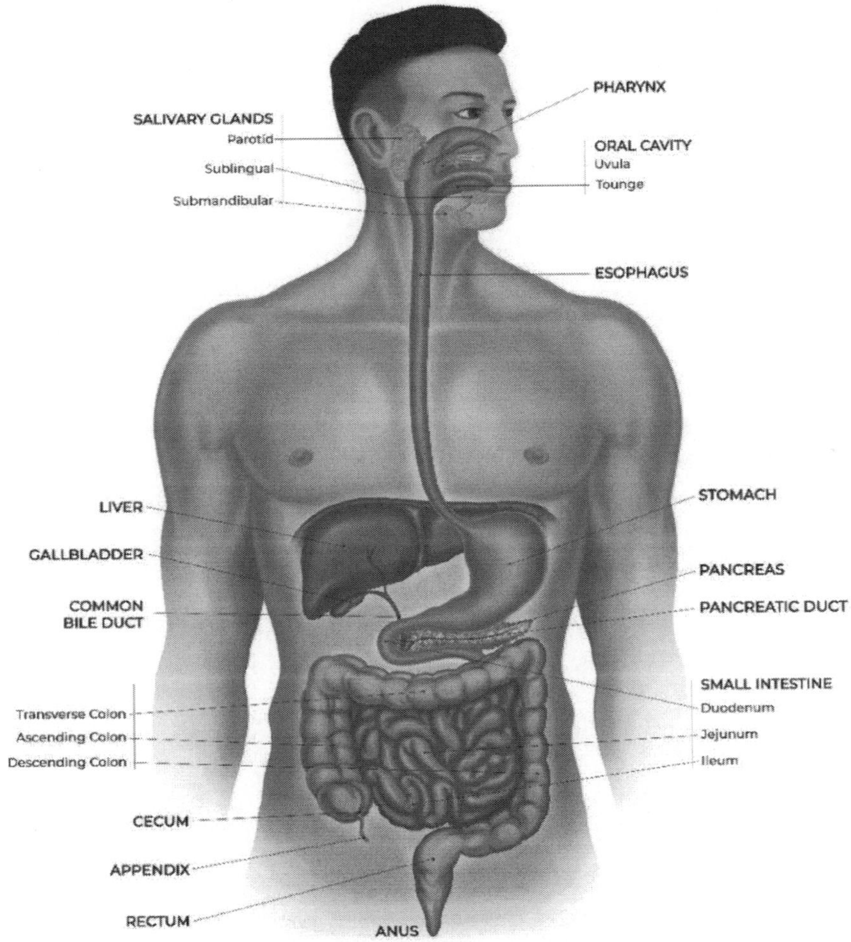

Peristalsis and Gastric Emptying

The gastrointestinal tract is a large muscle and **peristalsis** is the uniform movement and contraction of these muscles to push gastric contents down the gastrointestinal tract. As food moves, it causes the gastrointestinal tract to stretch and this causes the muscles behind the food to contract and the muscles in front of the food to relax. This coordinated contraction and relaxation moves the food downward at a speed that allows nutrients to be absorbed in the proper location. Gastrointestinal muscle is enervated by the sympathetic and parasympathetic system and as such sympathetic stimulus will decrease peristalsis and parasympathetic stimulus will increase peristalsis. Movement of gastric contents through the pyloric sphincter and into the small intestine is regulated simultaneously by peristaltic contractions and how much the pyloric sphincter opens to allow passing of gastric contents. A large amount of chyme in the stomach will cause the pyloric sphincter to open larger to allow more chyme to pass through.

Biomacromolecules

Formation of Micelles

Lipid molecules contain both long non-polar hydrophobic hydrocarbon tails and polar hydrophilic head groups. Naturally, a group of lipids will coagulate into **micelles** in an aqueous solution. A typical micelle is often a spherical formation of lipid aggregates, with the hydrophilic polar heads grouped in direct contact with the aqueous solvent, while the non-polar hydrocarbon tails are protected within the micelle sphere, sequestering any interaction the tails might have with the solvent. Reverse micelles can also occur, with the polar head sequestered in the center, while the hydrocarbon tails extend outward toward the solvent, as in the case of water drops in a cup of oil. Lipid bilayers are a specialized type of micelle that allows for a proper enclosed membrane to form, thus allowing cells to survive and flourish.

Classes of Carbohydrates

The **four class of carbohydrates** are as follows:

- **Monosaccharide**: The simplest form of sugar, a singular molecule, e.g., Glucose, galactose and fructose.
- **Disaccharides**: The binding of two monosaccharide subunits, e.g., sucrose: glucose-fructose, maltose: glucose-glucose, lactose: glucose-galactose.
- **Oligosaccharides**: Generally consist of three to ten monosaccharide subunits bound together, e.g., fructo-oligosaccharides (FOS) and insulins.
- **Polysaccharides**: Generally consists of ten or more monosaccharides subunits. Polysaccharides can be broken down further into two separate categories:
- ***Homopolysaccharides***: Polysaccharide that contains the same monosaccharide subunits. (e.g., starch, glycogen, cellulose)
- ***Heteropolysaccharide***: Polysaccharide that contains more than one type of monosaccharide subunit, i.e. heteroglycan.

Glycogen Synthesis and Glycogen Degradation

Glucose is taken up by the cell and converted to glucose-6-phosphate. Glucose-6-phosphate can be converted to energy through glycolysis, or it can be converted to glycogen. Glycogen is a branched polysaccharide of glucose and acts as a temporary storage of glucose. During **glycogen synthesis,** glucose-6-phosphate is converted to glucose-1-phosphate. Glucose -1-phosphate is converted with the addition of uridine triphosphate (UTP, similar to ATP), to UDP-Glucose. Glycogen synthase binds the UDP-Glucose to the glycogen molecule, elongating the glycogen molecule, releasing the UDP molecule. While glycogen synthase elongates an existing glycogen molecule, it cannot initiate the creation of a new molecule. A new glycogen molecule is synthesized by a glucose molecule binding to the active site of the glycogenin enzyme. Glycogen synthase is regulated and activated hormonally by glucagon. **Glycogen degradation** occurs often during heavy exercise or the fight/flight response and is regulated by epinephrine (adrenalin). Glycogen degradation is mediated by glycogen phosphorylase.

Structures of Protein Organization

The following are the four **structures of protein organization**:

- **Primary structure**: Amino acid sequence and covalent bond location within a polypeptide chain of a protein.
- **Secondary structure**: Local folding of the primary structure or polypeptide chains of the protein in response between stabilizing hydrogen bonds and polar amino acid side chains, which can give rise to specific geometrical shapes: α helix, β sheet, or U-turns.
- **Tertiary structure**: Is the overall conformation of the polypeptide chain that is stabilized by hydrophobic interactions between nonpolar amino acid side chains as well as disulfide bonds, rather than hydrogen bonds. Within this three-dimensional scaffold, the secondary structures are stabilized.
- **Quaternary structure**: Describes when two monomeric proteins (singular proteins that have adopted tertiary structures) bind usually through covalent bonds, to form a dimeric protein.

Simple Proteins and Conjugated Proteins

Simple proteins are the most basic class of proteins that when hydrolyzed and broken down, the byproducts of the degradation are amino acids only such as histones, albumin, and globulins. **Conjugated proteins** are a class of proteins that function through interaction with non-amino prosthetic groups. When hydrolyzed, these proteins will provide amino acids as well as various prosthetic groups, which could include carbohydrates, lipids, nucleic acids, phosphates, and metal ions. Examples of conjugated proteins include glycoproteins (mucin), chromoproteins/hemoproteins (hemoglobin), lipoproteins (Low density lipoproteins, LDL), nucleoproteins (nuclein), phosphoproteins (calcineurins) and metaloproteins.

Essential and Non-Essential Amino Acids

An **essential amino acid** is an amino acid that cannot be synthesized by mammals and must be obtained by other means, through diet or dietary supplements. Examples of essential amino acids include:

- Phenylalanine (Phe, F)
- Leucine (Leu, L)
- Methionine (Met, M)
- Lysine (Lys, K)
- Isoleucine (Ile, I)
- Valine (Val, V)
- Threonine (Thr, T)
- Tryptophan (Trp, W)
- Histidine (His, H)
- Arginine (Arg, R)

Non-essential amino acids are amino acids that are normally synthesized by mammals. Supplements may be used in cases of deficiency. Examples of non-essential amino acids include:

- Alanine (Ala, A)
- Asparagine (Asn, N)
- Aspartate (Asp, D)
- Cysteine (Cys, C)
- Glutamate (Glu, E)
- Glutamine (Gln, Q)
- Glycine (Gly, G)
- Proline (Pro, P)
- Serine (Ser, S)
- Tyrosine (Tyr, Y)

Theories of Acid/Base

The Arrhenius theory, Bronsted-Lowry theory, and Lewis Electronic theory are explained below:

- **Arrhenius theory**: The acid is a molecule or ion that releases hydrogen ions (H+) into the solution and a base is a molecule that releases hydroxyl ions (OH-).
- **Bronsted—Lowry theory**: An acid is a molecule or ion that donates protons, while base is a molecule that accepts protons.

- **Lewis Electronic theory**: Indicates that an acid is a molecule or an ion that creates a covalent bond by accepting a pair of electrons from base. A base, however, has a pair of unshared electrons, which can be donated to an acid to create a covalent bond.

The strength of an acid depends on how easily and readily a molecule can release hydrogen ions, protons, or accept unshared electrons from a base. The strength of a base depends on how readily a molecule donates electron pairs, releases hydroxyl ions, or accepts a proton from an acid.

Enzymology

ENZYME KINETICS

Enzyme kinetics is the study of how enzymes (usually protein molecules although also RNA molecules) catalyze (cause) chemical reactions. Kinetics refers both to how reactions occur and to the rates of reactions. Enzymes have active sites to which target/reactant substrate molecules bind, resulting in transformation of the substrate in a number of steps (enzymatic mechanism). The substrates may interact with the protein after they bind in order to facilitate binding in a process referred to as induced fit to improve the reaction. Some enzymes bind to one target molecule and others to multiple. Different types of reactions may occur: Some substrates become multiple products and others combine to form a larger or different molecule. The rate of reaction may vary according to different factors. For example, reaction rates may increase as temperature increases although excessively high temperature may result in denaturing (loss of shape and activity) of the enzyme. Changes in pH may also affect reactivity. At the end of the reaction, the enzyme releases any products of the reaction.

ENZYMES

Enzyme	Function
Ligase	Enzymes that catalyze two molecules or DNA fragments to allow them to bond chemically, such as DNA ligase. These enzymes have an important role in the replication and repair of DNA.
Hydrolase	Includes 200+ hydrolytic enzymes that catalyze water to divide molecules. Includes esterases, lipases, proteases, nucleosidases, and glucosidases.
Transferase	Includes 450+ different enzymes (such as transaminase) that catalyze the transfer of non-hydrogen chemical groups from a donor molecule to a recipient molecule. (The transfer of hydrogen atoms and electrons is catalyzed by dehydrogenases/oxidases.)
Isomerase	Enzyme that catalyzes the transformation of a chemical compound/molecule from one isomer into another. (An isomer is a molecule with the same formula as another but with different atomic structure and properties).
Kinase	Enzyme that transfers phosphate groups from a phosphate-donating molecule (such as adenosine triphosphate) to a substrate in a process called phosphorylation as part of regulation of cell function.

Digestive Enzymes

Enzyme	Function
Amylase	Produced in the pancreas and glands of the small intestinal mucosa and in saliva. Converts carbohydrates (starch) into dextrin, maltose, and glucose by catalyzing hydrolysis.
Lipase (Pharyngeal)	Produced in the pharyngeal mucosa. Converts triglycerides into fatty acids, diglycerides, and monoglycerides.
Lipase (Pancreatic)	Produced in the pancreas. Converts triglycerides into fatty acids, diglycerides, and monoglycerides as part of fat digestion.
Protease	Produced in the pancreas and released into the small intestine. Enzymes that catalyze the peptide bonds of amino acids to breakdown proteins. Proteases have a role in many body processes, such as blood clotting, immune response, replication of DNA, and cell proliferation/differentiation.

Processes of Metabolism

Metabolism can be broken down into two processes: catabolism and anabolism. **Catabolism** involves the breaking down of larger macromolecules into small smaller subunits for the main purpose of energy production. Larger macromolecules can also be broken down into smaller subunits to allowing for easier excretion through urine or feces. Additionally, smaller subunits from larger macromolecules can be recycled and reused, such as amino acid subunits from protein. Important pathways of catabolism include glycolysis, the citric acid cycle (Krebs cycle), and the electron transport chain or oxidative phosphorylation, which through the break down of glucose provides a net gain of energy through production of adenosine triphosphate (ATP) by means of phosphorylation of adenosine diphosphate (ADP). Catabolism drives the anabolism process. **Anabolism** involves the production of large macromolecules from simpler subunits through the hydrolysis of ATP to ADP. Anabolism pathways include DNA replication, translation, transcription and glycogen synthesis.

Energy Yield in Aerobic Metabolism vs. Anaerobic Metabolism

In **aerobic metabolism** glucose is broken down by glycolysis to form pyruvate, which is then converted to acetyl CoA, and further broken down in the citric acid cycle, and by the electron transport chain (oxidative phosphorylation) providing energy formation as adenosine triphosphate (ATP). Glycolysis provides a net gain of two ATP. The citric acid cycle and electron transport chain provide a theoretical net gain of 36 ATP. However, the actual ATP produced per glucose molecule is closer to 30. ATP is the energy source that fuels the majority of the intracellular tasks necessary for life. With anaerobic metabolism, the citric acid cycle and electron transport chain are bypassed, and glucose is only broken down by glycolysis. The cells sacrifice the amount of ATP formed for speed by which the glucose is broken down. The glucose is broken down in glycolysis leading to a net gain of 2 ATP. Anaerobic metabolism is necessary for strenuous muscle work.

Cori Cycle

During heavy exercise, muscles adopt anaerobic metabolism, uncoupling glycolysis from the citric acid cycle, and oxidative phosphorylation, converting glucose into lactic acid. Lactic acid builds up in the muscle, leading to a burning aching sensation when used heavily. The lactic acid diffuses from the muscle into the circulation. The lactic acid is absorbed by the liver, and converted into glucose, which is released into the blood, providing more energy for the muscles. This cycle known as the **Cori cycle,** provides a means by which the body can maintain muscle activity under anaerobic conditions, which is vital for the fight or flight response as well as important in strenuous exercise.

Purine Synthesis

Biosynthesis pathways of the purine nucleotides lead to the formation of an activated sugar subgroup, known as 5-phosphoribosyl-1-pyrophosphate (PPRP). PPRP is the beginning subunit for all nucleotide synthesis as well as the beginning subunit for salvage or recycling of nucleotide subunits. **Synthesis of purine nucleotides** occurs mainly in the liver. PPRP undergoes several enzymatic reactions to be converted into inosine 5'-monophosphate (IMP). IMP acts as the basis of the purine nucleotides and can be converted into either adenine (A) or guanine nucleotide (G), depending on levels of GTP and ATP respectively. The conversion of IMP to AMP is facilitated by the energy from GTP and the opposite is true when GMP is biosynthesized. This allows for a check and balance to occur within the cells for purine synthesis, if GTP levels are in excess, then AMP synthesis will flourish. If ATP levels are in excess, GMP synthesis will flourish.

Partial and Full Agonists and Antagonists

An **agonist** is a ligand that can activate a particular receptor. A **partial agonist** is a ligand that activates a receptor below full activity. **Co-agonists** are two or more ligands that bind, leading to the activation of the receptor. Partial agonists can also be considered as **partial antagonists**, or ligands that lead to partial inhibition of the receptor. **Full antagonists** lead to full inhibition.

Competitive and Non-Competitive Inhibition

There are two types of inhibition, competitive inhibition and noncompetitive inhibition. **Competitive inhibition** occurs when the antagonist competes with the agonist at the binding region of the receptor. This form of inhibition is reversible. Adding higher concentrations of the agonist can displace the antagonist, returning receptor activity to normal. **Noncompetitive inhibition** occurs when an antagonist binds to a region of the receptor that leads to a conformational change of the protein, so that the agonist cannot activate the receptor. Noncompetitive inhibition is irreversible and usually the receptor must be sequestered by the cell and replaced before the agonist can activate the receptor again.

Cell Chemistry

Roles of Organelles

Described below are the roles of organelles:

- **Cell membrane**: A semi-permeable phospholipid bilayer, which acts as a physical barrier between the intracellular components of a cell and the extracellular environment. It is an important mediator of signaling due to the semi-permeable membrane and important signaling/transport proteins.
- **Rough endoplasmic reticulum (rER):** Network of membranes interconnected with the nuclear envelope. The surface of the rER is covered with ribosomes. The rER is important in the translation of proteins that are to be excreted from the cell or placed in the cellular membrane.
- **Smooth endoplasmic reticulum**: Similar to the rER, but lacks the ribosomes. It is important in detoxification and serves as a store of calcium, necessary for intracellular signaling.
- **Mitochondria**: A membrane bound organelle. It contains two membranes. Within the mitochondria; the citric acid cycle and oxidative phosphorylation occurs, important final steps in the breakdown of glucose that leads to ATP formation, the energy of the cell.

- **Lysosome organelles**: Important in the digestion of food, organelles, bacteria and viruses. Digestive enzymes are held in an enclosed vacuole, away from the intracellular workings of the cell.

Cell Cycle

Cells spend the majority of their lifespan in the **G1 phase** of the cell cycle. It lies in between **mitosis** and the **S phase**. During the G1 phase, nutrients are absorbed and cellular activity and cell size increase. The S phase occurs when cells have begun to synthesize and replicate the DNA chromosomes. The **G2 phase** is a period of rapid cellular growth that occurs in preparation of the final stage of cellular replication, mitosis. The G1, S, and G2 phases can be lumped into the phase known as the **interphase of the growth cycle**.

Mitosis (M phase) consists of four important stages.

1. **Prophase**: DNA condenses into sister chromosomes bound together at the centromere. Formation of the microtubule chromatins occurs as well as nuclear envelope breakdown.
2. **Metaphase**: Microtubule chromatins bind to centromere complex and aid in the alignment of chromosomes across the central plane of the cell.
3. **Anaphase**: Microtubule chromatins shorten, pulling sister chromatids apart toward opposite ends of the cell.
4. **Telophase/cytokinesis**: Nuclear envelope reforms, chromatins unwind, cytoplasm increases and cells divide.

Steps of Meiosis

Meiosis is how diploid cells divide into haploid cells, forming important reproductive cells (gametes) such as sperm and eggs. Meiosis consists of two cell divisions. Everything before the cell divisions into the gametes is known as interphase, which includes DNA synthesis.

- **Prophase I**: Replicated DNA condenses into chromosomes, with two sister chromatids bound to each other. The nuclear envelope disappears.
- **Metaphase I**: Homologous chromosome pairs are lined up at the central plane by polar microtubule centrioles.
- **Anaphase I**: Microtubules shorten, pulling apart homologous chromosomes, sister chromatids remain together.
- **Telophase I**: Two daughter cells are formed with half the amount of DNA in each cell, but chromosomes that are still present are in sister chromatids. Prophase II, new centrioles form and sister chromatids begin to move toward the central plane of the cell.
- **Metaphase II**: The chromatids are aligned in the central plane of the cell.
- **Anaphase II**: Sister chromatids are pulled apart toward opposite ends of the cell, as microtubule centrioles shorten.
- **Telophase II**: Nuclear envelope changes, cytokinesis occurs giving four separate gamete cells from one original parental cell.

Apoptosis vs. Necrosis

Cells generally undergo two types of death, apoptosis and necrosis. **Apoptosis** is an evolutionarily conserved programmed cell death. Apoptosis occurs in individual cells in response to various intracellular and extracellular signals, which lead to the activation of specific proteases that begin to degrade important cellular components. Common signs of apoptosis are the creation of apoptotic body, specific cleavage of the DNA, integrity of the membrane is maintained, and release of important mitochondrial enzymes. Apoptosis is an active form of cell death, requiring the use of energy (ATP) to proceed. It can be caused by physiological and pathological injuries and is generally considered a "clean" death. **Necrosis** is generally caused only by pathological injury. Necrosis is a passive cell death, does not require energy. Necrosis is not regulated; DNA is not cleaved, the membrane loses its integrity as the cells burst, leaking the intracellular components into the extracellular matrix. Necrosis deals with injury of tissue more than individual cells. Necrotic cells are removed by macrophages.

Chemical Bonds

A chemical bond is the attraction of atoms to form simple and complex molecules.

- **Covalent bonds** are the strong bonds that occur through the sharing of electrons between atoms. Covalent bonds can occur as single bonds, double bonds, or triple bonds.
- An ion is an atom that has gained or lost an electron, becoming a cation (+) or anion (-). **Ionic bonds** occur through the attraction of oppositely charged ions and can form between atoms, creating strong crystal-like structures such as NaCl (table salt).
- When hydrogen binds to an electronegative atom, the hydrogen adopts a weak positive charge while the electronegative atom such as chloride adopts a slight negative charge, creating a dipole molecule. The positively charged hydrogen creates a weak bond with electronegative atoms of another molecule. **Hydrogen bonds** help form the structure of DNA and proteins. Van der Waals forces are also known as intramolecular forces, which are very weak overall attractive and repulsive properties of molecules to other molecules in gas or liquid.

Autocrine, Paracrine, Synaptic, and Endocrine Signaling

Autocrine signaling is the self-stimulation of cells by a signaling molecule such as a growth factor. **Paracrine signaling** is the stimulation of target cells by a signaling molecule produced by local adjacent cells. **Synaptic signaling** is a form of paracrine signaling that is specific to neurons. Signaling of nerve cells often occurs by the release of neurotransmitters from the synapse to other cells which can lead to important physiological changes. **Endocrine signaling** is the systematic signaling of hormones released by endocrine glands throughout the body.

Ion Channels

Ion channels are an important in regulating electrical chemical gradients across a cell, which has important roles in the nerve system, cardiac system, and is also important in maintenance of the osmotic gradient. Ions generally flow from a higher gradient to a lower gradient and can have very important roles with local cellular signaling as well as systematic signaling (hormones, active potentials). Ion channels are imbedded in the membrane and show high selectivity toward specific ions (i.e. Na+, K+, Ca2+). Ion channels can be always open, allowing free flow of ions into a cell and down the concentration gradient, which is often linked to the transport of other molecules into a cell, even if against its concentration gradient. Ion channels can also be voltage dependent, opening in response to changes in the electric membrane potential. These types of ions are important in propagating a signal such as an action potential in a nerve cell. Ion channels that do not function properly can give rise to many disorders such as epilepsy and migraines.

Endocytosis and Exocytosis

Endocytosis is the process by which vesicles are formed from the cell membrane of a cell and molecules from the extracellular fluid are taken into the cell. Many molecules that a cell requires are polar in nature and therefore require the process of endocytosis to get across the hydrophobic cell membrane. Pinocytosis is a special type of endocytosis that occurs when only extracellular fluid is taken into the cell. Phagocytosis is the other type of endocytosis that is specific to small molecules being taken up by the cell. In phagocytosis, molecules must first bind to a specific cell membrane receptor, which then signals the cell to form a vesicle to bring the molecule into the cell. **Exocytosis** is functionally the opposite of endocytosis and is used most often for a cell to release proteins, enzymes, and hormones into the extracellular space. Exocytosis is vital for the process of cellular signaling to occur.

Endosymbiotic Theory

The endosymbiotic theory attempts to explain the origin of mitochondria and chloroplasts, an important component of eukaryotic cells. Mitochondria via the electron can synthesize ATP, a necessary energy for the cell. Chloroplasts can use sunlight to aid in the synthesis of ATP. Mitochondria and chloroplasts resemble bacteria in many ways, including the presence of their own circular DNA molecules. Also, although mitochondrial and chloroplast replication is regulated by the eukaryotic cells, their replication in many ways is separate and resemble replication of a bacteria. It is thought that larger cells, at one point, engulfed smaller bacteria, but did not phagocytose these cells, creating instead a symbiotic relationship that allowed safety for the smaller bacteria and energy for the larger cells. As evolution progressed, the larger and smaller cells became more dependent on each other and soon gave rise to the first eukaryotic cells.

Reproduction of Mitochondria

Mitochondrial pathways are regulated by proteins translated, not only by nuclear mRNA, and are also regulated by mitochondrial DNA. Mitochondrial DNA resembles DNA found in bacteria, a circular molecule of DNA. Mitochondrial DNA codes for several proteins involved in the electron transport chain, ATP production as well as protein synthesis. Replication is dependent on energy needs of the cell rather than the cell cycle. Mitochondria replicate in a way similar to binary fission, a form of asexual reproduction used by bacteria. Generally occurring after DNA replication and cell growth, the sister circular chromosomes separate to polar ends of the growing cell, similar to mitosis and cytokinesis occurs, providing two identical daughter mitochondria.

Angiogenesis and Vasculogenesis

Biologically, vasculogenesis and angiogenesis are very similar in that they both regulate growth of blood vessels. **Vasculogenesis** is essential during embryogenesis, regulating the development of blood vessels in response to various signaling cues. Vasculogenesis is generally thought of as spontaneous blood vessel formation, while angiogenesis regulates growth of blood vessels from already existing blood vessels. Many of the signaling cues between angiogenesis and vasculogenesis overlap. Both angiogenesis and vasculogenesis are important in development. **Angiogenesis** also has important roles in wound repair. The process of angiogenesis is manipulated by tumors. Many tumors, once they reach a certain size, cannot maintain their growth through normal diffusion, they need a blood supply. By expressing common protein inducers of angiogenesis, such as vascular endothelial growth factor (VEGF), the tumors can direct angiogenesis and blood vessel formation. These new blood vessels can integrate into the tumor, bringing necessary nutrients so the tumor and cancer can survive.

Passive Cellular Transport Mechanisms and Active Transport

The four main passive cellular transport mechanisms and active transport are discussed below:

- **Diffusion**: Involves moving any molecule from an area of higher concentration to an area of lower concentration.
- **Filtration**: Similar to diffusion, however, filtration moves gasses and fluids from higher to lower pressure areas.

- **Osmosis**: A type of diffusion that is specifically related to water moving back and forth between a membrane that is permeable to water. In this case, water moves from higher to lower areas of concentration due entirely to a difference in particle number on each side of the membrane. Water will continue to move until the particle number is equal on both sides of the membrane.
- **Conduction**: In conduction, ions become susceptible to various positive and negative forces that are produced in an electrical field. In this case, positive ions will move away from an area with a large positive charge and negative ions will move away from an area with a large negative charge.
- **Active Transport**: Involves using energy to move anything against any type of gradient. This is accomplished with the use of a variety of transmembrane proteins.

DNA/RNA

Conservative and Semi-Conservative Models of DNA Replication

Originally there were two proposed **models for how DNA replicates** either conservative or semi-conservative replication.

- The proposed hypothesis for **conserved replication** stated that a completely new chromosome with new DNA base pairs would be created, using the older original chromosome as a template. This replication model did not hold true.
- **Semi-conservative replication** occurs when two chromosome copies are replicated, with each new chromosome containing one DNA strand from the original chromosome. The semi-conservative model for DNA replication has shown to be true for DNA replication in all eukaryotic and prokaryotic cell types.

Nucleotides in DNA and RNA

Nucleotides contain three parts, a deoxyribose sugar, phosphate group, and a nitrogenous base. There are two types of nucleotide classes: pyrimidines and purines. Adenine (A) and guanine (G) are purines, while thymidine (T), cytosine (C) and uracil (U) are pyrimidines. Nucleotides make up the structure of DNA and RNA. The backbone structure of the molecule is the deoxyribose sugar. Base pairs bind to each other in a single strand through a phosphodiester bond between the 5' and 3' hydroxyl groups of the bases. Due to this configuration, DNA and RNA must replicate in the orientation from the 5' to the 3' end. Four bases are found in DNA: A,G,C,T. It is the base pairs that encode the important genes for our life. Through hydrogen bonding A will bind to T, and G will bind to C, allowing the proper structure of the DNA to form. This type of bonding also allows for easy separation of the strands during replication and RNA synthesis. In RNA, thymidine is replaced by uracil. Generally, RNA is single stranded with important roles in protein synthesis.

Creating Recombinant DNA Pharmaceuticals from Ligated cDNA and Genomic DNA

mRNA can be extracted from tissue and cells, and using an enzyme known as **reverse transcriptase**, the mRNA can be converted into cDNA, a DNA copy of the mRNA strand. This cDNA can be used to amplify a specific human gene, which can encode for an important protein, by using the biological technique known as Polymerase chain reaction. The cDNA copy, after using specific restriction enzymes, can be inserted into a DNA vector. DNA ligase is used to seal the new gene into the vector, stabilizing it. The vector usually contains an antibiotic resistant gene (i.e. ampicillin), which when transfected into bacteria, only bacteria with this vector will be able to live on the antibiotic. The bacteria colony with the correct vector will be grown. The amplified vector is purified and sterility is checked. If everything appears sound it can be used in future experiments, or in the case of medicine, can be formulated properly/ packaged and a recombinant DNA pharmaceutical can be created. In a similar fashion, using specific restriction enzymes, genomic DNA can be cleaved and ligated into a vector, amplified and purified similar to a cDNA vector.

Electroporation

Electroporation is a technique that uses an electrical field that is applied to cells to increase the chance of transfection of recombinant DNA/RNA plasmids into the cells. Electroporation increases cell permeability by causing transient pores to form in the plasma membrane. If short enough, the introduction of the electrical field will allow the cells to take up the plasmid, the pores will close, and the cell will survive. If too long, the cells will die. This type of transfection will lead to a high percentage of transfection although there is also a high level of cell death. If cultured properly, the surviving cells will grow and the new colony will possess the plasmid, and a stable cell culture will be created.

Forms of RNA

The following are the most common forms of RNA found in cells:

- **Ribosomal RNA or rRNA**: The most abundant form of RNA found in the cell, rRNA is an important component of the ribosome, which plays a vital role during translation and protein synthesis. Approximately 80% of cellular RNA is made up of rRNA.
- **Messenger RNA or mRNA**: During transcription, complement RNA copies of DNA are created, which allows the message in the genes of the DNA to be carried to cytosol by mRNA for specific protein synthesis. Approximately 5% of cellular RNA is made up of mRNA
- **Transfer RNA or tRNA**: tRNA carries specific amino acids necessary for protein synthesis. By binding to a codon region (a specific three-base pair region on mRNA), with a complementary anticodon region on the tRNA (to ensure proper binding), tRNA can facilitate lengthening of the amino acid sequence of the protein during synthesis. Approximately 15% of all cellular RNA is tRNA.

Microorganisms

Classification of Viruses

Viruses (virions) are sub-microscopic and generally considered non-living because they lack cell structures. Viruses consist of nucleic acid, single or double-strand DNA and/or RNA (the genome), encapsulated in a protein coating called a capsid. Some have a lipid envelope about the capsid with glycoprotein spikes. The purpose of viruses is to reproduce, but they require a host cell with a protein receptor to which a virus must bind to penetrate the cell membrane. The viral genome carries encoding that allows it to use the cell to replicate in a lytic or lysogenic cycle. In the lytic cycle, the virus forces the cell to manufacture proteins and new genomes. After new viral particles form, the cell ruptures, releasing the viruses. In a lysogenic cycle, the virus integrates the DNA of the host and as the cell replicates, the virus replicates with it. The virus remains dormant until it activates and begins a lytic cycle. Viruses that infect bacteria are bacteriophages (or phages). Retroviruses are a sub-category of viruses. Retroviruses must have 3 characteristics: a genome that contains ribonucleic acid (RNA), the enzyme reverse transcriptase, and a protein body surrounding by a protein envelope. While some viruses contain DNA, retroviruses do not.

Classification of Bacteria

Bacteria are critical for human survival and while most are benign, some are pathogenic, leading to infection. Bacteria are ubiquitous, with about 10 times as many bacteria in the human body as there are human cells. Bacteria have simple prokaryote structures, with no membrane-encased nucleus or organelles but a tangle of looped DNA called a nucleoid. Bacteria also have plasmids, which are double strands of DNA outside of the nucleoid that allow for transmission from cell to cell or by attaching to viruses. Essentially, bacteria are able to trade genes, making them very adaptable. The cell membrane of most bacteria, except the Mollicutes (mycoplasmas), is surrounded by a cell wall, the composition of which varies. It's the composition of this cell wall that determines the Gram-staining, either negative or positive. Bacteria have 4 different shapes:

- Cocci (round), occur in chains or clusters (Staphylococci, Streptococci, Diplococci).
- Spiral, includes spirillum (*Campylobacter* spp, *Helicobacter* spp) and spirochetes (*Treponema pallidum, Borrelia* spp).
- Bacilli (rods), occur singly, doubly, or in filaments.
- Incomplete spirals (*Vibrio* spp).

Classification of Fungi

Fungi were originally classified as plants, but they do not produce their own food through photosynthesis and must, like animals, get the food from another source. Fungi vary widely, from one-celled microorganisms to multi-celled chains that are miles long. Fungi are used to make antibiotics, but they can also cause infection and disease. Two common classifications of fungi are molds (including mushrooms) and yeast. Fungi are not motile, but some produce spores, which can be inhaled. Some, such as the yeast *Candida albicans*, are part of the normal flora of the skin but can overgrow in an opportunistic infection. As microorganisms, fungal infections can invade the sinuses, the mouth, the respiratory system, and the vagina. Antibiotics may affect the balance between bacteria and yeast, causing infection. Fungal infections include histoplasmosis, blastomycosis, and coccidioidomycosis. Fungal infections, such as *Pneumocystis jiroveci (*formerly *carinii)* pose a serious problem for the immunocompromised. Antifungal drugs are available, but systemic fungal infections are difficult to treat.

Classification of Protozoa

Protozoa are single-cell microorganisms with a nucleus that live primarily off of bacteria. They share similarities to animals, but (except for Myxozoa) they are not, and they are also not plants. Many protozoa are free living and are ubiquitous in soil and water. They are often divided according to their method of locomotion: flagellates, amoeboids, sporozoans, and ciliates. Some protozoa are able to form protective cysts, which can survive outside the host, sometimes for long periods, before transmission to another host. Protozoa are parasites to humans and cause a wide range of infections. Enteric protozoa, such as *Giardia intestinalis* and *Entamoeba histolytica,* can cause severe diarrhea. Other diseases caused by protozoa include malaria, Chagas disease, babesiosis, toxoplasmosis, trichomonas infection, and amoebic dysentery. Protozoa take a huge toll of life, especially in developing countries, but some diseases, such as Chagas disease, or becoming more common in the United States as people emigrate from endemic areas of Latin America.

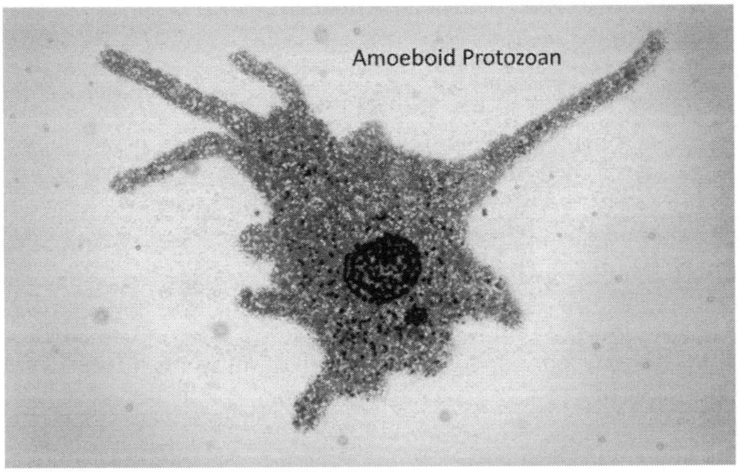

Classification of Algae

Algae, in the family Protista, include a large number of primarily aquatic (fresh or salt water) organisms that contain chlorophyll, and most utilize photosynthesis to manufacture food (autotrophic growth) although some flourish in the dark by using starches (heterotrophic growth). Algae may have plant-like or animal-like characteristics or a combination of both. Algae include some that are multicellular (such as seaweed and giant kelp) and many single-cell forms (such as cyanobacteria, which is similar to bacteria). Common types of algae include diatoms (fresh water), dinoflagellates (salt water) red algae (seaweeds), green algae (plantlike), and brown algae (kelp). Algae have an important role in the production of oxygen, producing 70% to 80% of atmospheric oxygen, as the process of photosynthesis results in the release of oxygen. Algae also provide the base of the aquatic food chain.

Classification of Archaea

Archaea were originally classified as bacteria and known as archaebacteria but in 1977 were reclassified. Archaea are single-cell prokaryotic organisms (lacking defined nucleus) that are distinct from bacteria and eukaryotic organisms. They can be found in many shapes (rod, spherical, irregular, rectangular) and may live alone or in filaments or clusters. Archaea are most commonly found in extreme environments, such as at high temperatures in hydrothermal vents and hot springs and in extremely acidic or alkaline environments. They also thrive in highly saline environments and are present in plankton. They survive in anaerobic environments, such as the gastrointestinal tract of animals (including humans), aiding in digestion and producing methane. Archaea are of special interest to scientists because of their ability to thrive in environments inhospitable to other organisms. Also, they can produce organic matter and energy from inorganic matter (ammonia, hydrogen).

Normal and Transient Flora

Normal flora are important colonies of bacteria in the body, often found in the gut, which at the very least do not cause disease, but more often have a symbiotic relationship with the host organism by aiding the host organism in proper digestion and nutrient absorption. Normal flora can also prevent growth of more dangerous bacteria. Normal flora can at times become overgrown, leading to disease, although this usually is rare. Bacteria and other microorganisms that cause disease are considered **transient flora**, which can infect the host organism for a time, before being removed by the immune system or treated with antibiotics or other therapy.

Gram Staining, Gram-Negative, and Gram-Positive Bacteria

Gram staining is a method created by Hans Christian Gram which helped divide bacteria species into two large subgroups, gram-negative or gram-positive, which are based on the chemical and physical characteristics of the bacterium's cell wall.

- **Gram-positive bacteria** have a cell wall that is thick with peptidoglycan, a polymer consisting of carbohydrates and amino acids, which will stain purple in the gram-stain test.
- **Gram negative bacteria** have a much thinner layer of peptidoglycan and tend to stain pink. Briefly, gram staining consists of only a few steps, including staining with crystal violet to a fixed bacterial colony, followed by a treatment of iodine, which fixes the crystal violet stain to the cells, and finally the bacteria are washed with ethanol.

Bacteria that stain positive will be a deep purple color, as mentioned above. Bacteria that are gram-negative will show no stain or will stain a very light pink color.

Microbial Genetics

Microbial genetics involves the study of the transfer of heritable information in microorganisms, including bacteria, archaea, fungi, protozoa, and viruses. Most research has focused on prokaryotic microorganisms, such as bacteria, which undergo different forms of recombination--general, site-specific, and replicative—as opposed to sexual reproduction that occurs with eukaryotic microorganisms (yeasts and other fungi). Microbes are utilized in the study of inheritance, gene structure, gene expression, gene regulation, and mutation. Reproduction and mutation rates are higher in microorganisms than in multicellular organisms, so study results are easier to obtain. DNA recombinant techniques are often utilized in studies of microbial genetics. Because inheritable processes with genetic material passed on through DNA are similar in microorganisms and multicellular organisms, these microorganisms can be studied to gain information about inheritance that can be applied to human beings. For example, assessing the degree to which the DNA in a microorganism mutates in response to an environmental toxin may help to determine risks to humans.

Pathogenic Microorganisms

UTIs

Microbials commonly associated with urinary tract infections (UTI) include:

- *Escherichia coli* (80% of UTI cases)
- Staphylococcus saprophyticus (5–15% of UTI cases)
- Proteus mirabilis/Klebsiella pneumonia (~5% if UTI cases)
- Other rare bacteria including Enterococcus, Pseudomonas and Neisseria gonorrhoeae can cause UTIs as well.

UTIs are often characterized as either lower (bladder infection) or upper (kidney infection). Symptoms include painful frequent urination, lower abdominal pain. Fever and chills also can be associated with UTIs. UTIs are more common in women than men. Pregnancy, recent sexual intercourse, history of infection can also increase the risk of UTIs. Treatment includes a short antibiotic course.

HEPATITIS

The route of infection, and symptoms for hepatitis (A, B, C) are as follows:

- **Hepatitis A** is an acute viral infection of the liver caused by H AV (Hepatitis A virus) and is generally transmitted through food that has been contaminated with fecal matter. It commonly occurs in people who use illegal drugs or who work in areas that are poorly hygienic. Symptoms include jaundice (yellowing of the skin), nausea, and abdominal pain.
- **Hepatitis B** causes liver inflammation. This disease is caused by HBV (hepatitis B virus) and is transmitted by blood transfusions, unprotected sex, and the use of dirty needles. Acute HBV infection symptoms are similar to hepatitis A. Chronic HBV infections can lead to a long-lasting inflammation of the liver which can lead to cirrhosis and cancer of the liver.
- **Hepatitis C** is transmitted by direct blood contact from an infected individual through blood transfusion, sharing of dirty needles, and sexual transmission. Acute hepatitis C symptoms will not manifest in most patients, but resemble symptoms observed in hepatitis A and B. Chronic hepatitis C leads to inflammation, cirrhosis and diabetes mellitus.

INFLUENZA

Influenza is also known as the flu. It is caused by an RNA virus. Common symptoms include fever, tiredness, respiratory distress, sore throat, muscle aches. The flu can lead to more serious disorders. The flu can be fatal, leading to nearly half a million deaths worldwide per year, or close to 40,000 deaths in the US. Treatment can include a yearly vaccine that can prevent the onset of the disease. Additionally, anti-influenza agents can be used for treatment. Amantadine and rimantadine inhibit replication of the virus by blocking removal of the viral coat, a necessity for replication. Zanamivir and oseltamivir are neuraminidase inhibitors. Neuraminidase is a viral protein necessary for release of the replicated virus from the infected cells, thus inhibiting further propagation of the virus.

HIV

Human immunodeficiency virus (HIV) is a retrovirus that can be transmitted by sexual intercourse or direct blood-to-blood contact with an infected person. HIV can also be transmitted from mother to the unborn fetus, although this transmission is rare, particularly if a caesarian section is performed during childbirth. HIV is an RNA retrovirus, which generally infects cells of the immune system including cd4 T-cells and macrophages. There are two main stages of HIV infection. The first stage occurs 2–4 weeks after exposure, in which the virus replicates incredibly fast, leading to a quick decline in CD4 T-cells. This stage appears similar to influenza. CD8 T-cells kill much of the infected T-cells, and the immune system removes the virus from the blood and CD4 cells return to a normal level. During this first stage, the disease is often misdiagnosed. The virus then enters a latent stage, which can remain latent for as long as twenty years. Over time, HIV leads to a decline of CD4 t-cells, which causes a decline in an effective immune system, and leads to the development of acquired immunodeficiency disease, in which the patients become susceptible to normally innocuous diseases.

CLOSTRIDIOIDES DIFFICILE

Clostridioides Difficile (C.Diff) is an anaerobic gram-positive bacterium that is very resistant to antibiotics. *C.Diff* adopts a rod shape that can release spores. *C.Diff* is considered normal flora of the intestines and is found in healthy individuals; however, it is also considered bad flora if it is ever allowed to grow unchecked leading to severe illness. Responses to disease, such as taking a lot of antibiotics to combat another infection, can lead to a decrease in the normal flora, allowing *C.Diff* to propagate and flourish. *C. Diff* can also be contagious through ingesting fecal matter. Also *C.Diff* creates spores that are extremely resistant and can be present for long periods of time in suboptimal growing environments. *C.Diff* generally causes damage to the intestinal wall, leading to lesions and ulcers in the intestines. *C.Diff* will initially cause abdominal pain and severe diarrhea. If the patient is not kept hydrated, this disease can be fatal. Treatment includes removal of antibiotics (if antibiotics are thought to be the cause) and the administration of metronidazole.

Sepsis and Septic Shock

Sepsis occurs in response to a severe systemic microbial infection. Sepsis is often associated with organ dysfunction and seems to occur as though the body is failing in response to the infection. Common symptoms of sepsis may include fever, rapid heart rate and hypoglycemia. Sepsis can progress and lead to septic shock, which occurs in response to multiple organ failure, decreased blood pressure, and decreased perfusion of oxygen into the tissue. Treatment can include broad-acting antimicrobial agents until the microbe that caused the infection is known. Such drugs as cefotaxime, cefepime, and ticarcillin-clavulanic acid have been indicated for treatment of sepsis. Corticosteroids and vasopressin are also indicated for treatment of sepsis and septic shock.

Emerging Infectious Diseases

An emerging infectious disease is an epidemic caused by infectious microbial organisms that show increased incidence levels from those observed in the past. Emerging infectious diseases can be relatively new diseases such as SARS, the avian flu, the West Nile virus, and Ebola virus. HIV, although it first emerged nearly thirty years ago, could be considered an emergent infectious agent. Also, other historical diseases such as tuberculosis, staph infections, smallpox and anthrax, which are showing or have the possibility of showing renewed incidence of the disease, can also be considered as emergent. Many causes can lead to an increased level of emergent diseases, such as the overuse of antimicrobial agents, which can lead to the formation of more drug-resistant microbials.

Microbiology Tests

Phenol Coefficient Test and Chick Martin Test

The **phenol coefficient test** is a standardized test to measure the effect of bactericidal compounds in relation to the bactericidal effects of phenol. Serial dilutions of the unknown bactericidal compound and phenol are performed in sterile tubes with cultured bacterial agents. The samples are inoculated for approximately ten minutes and then placed into fresh media and allowed to grow for a few more days. The highest dilutions of the compound that effectively killed the bacteria in that original ten minutes of the test are used to calculate the phenol coefficient which is calculated by:

Phenol coefficient = (1 – effective dose of Agent A)/(1 – effective dose of phenol)

The higher the coefficient, the greater the bactericidal effect of the unknown antibacterial agent.

The **chick-martin test** is a standardized test to measure the effect of anti-bacterial disinfectants in the presence of water and organic matter. The test uses serial dilutions of yeast and salmonella Typhi for thirty minutes. These compounds are tested compared to phenol and a phenol coefficient is determined similar to the above equation.

Acid Test

The **acid test stain** is an experimental test to study the presence of mycobacterium which can cause diseases such as tuberculosis. The collected components (sputum, blood, urine, bone marrow, organ biopsies, etc.) are placed on the slide and then stained. The bacteria are fixed by heating and the stain is rinsed with an acid wash and then counter-stained with another stain. Microorganisms that keep the original stain are known as acid-fast positive microorganisms. Being acid-fast positive is a common trait and indicator of mycobacterium infections.

Schick Test and the PPD Test

The **Schick test** was developed as a means to determine which people are susceptible to diphtheria. 0.1 mL of 1:150 dilution of the diphtheria toxin is injected via an intradermal route of administration, just below the skin. If a person does not have antibodies against diphtheria, the injection will become red and swollen for a couple days. If the person does have antibodies against diphtheria, there will be no reaction to the injected toxin. **PPD** test is also known as the Mantoux test or the tuberculin sensitivity test. The PPD test is a diagnostic tool to determine if someone has been infected with mycobacterium which can cause the disease tuberculosis. The test injects a low level of tuberculin, a protein extracted from mycobacterium. People exposed to mycobacterium will react to the tuberculin leading to redness and swelling. People who have not been exposed to tuberculin will show little or no reaction. A positive result needs to be evaluated by a physician to determine the significance of the reaction.

KOH Test

The **potassium hydroxide (KOH) test** is used to measure the presence of fungal infections on skin and nails, particularly infections caused by dermatophytes and *Candida Albicans* fungi. A few cells are collected from the skin or nails, usually by gentle scraping. The scraping is usually performed over a glass slide. KOH is added at a 1:10 dilution in water. The glass slide is heated and then stained with a blue dye. The KOH dissolves all the tissue that is not the fungus, while the dye stains and adds color to the fungi cells for easier visibility. The slide is viewed by light microscopy and if present, the fungi will show up, stained blue. If the slide is negative, nothing will be stained, as everything will be dissolved by the KOH.

Immunology

Active and Passive Immunity

Active immunity occurs when the immune system increases the production of antibodies against a foreign agent such as an infectious disease like influenza or due to administration of a vaccine against an antigen of a disease such as diphtheria. Active immunity is considered to be permanent. **Passive immunity**, unlike active immunity, diminishes over time. It occurs through transfer of antibodies from one person to another and generally only lasts a few weeks to a few months. Prime examples of passive immunity are antibodies that are transferred from a mother to a fetus in-utero as well as after birth through the mothers' milk.

Primary and Secondary Immune Responses

The **primary immune response** occurs when an antigen is first contacted by the immune system. Initially the response is slow; very few antibodies will be able to react with the antigen. This lag time in response is enough time for an antigen to cause sickness in the patient. During this time, B cells are making antibodies against the antigen to combat the infection. After the infection, the antibody levels decrease in the body. If the same antigen infects the host, memory of the previous infection still exists within the immune cells, and a **secondary response** is much more rapid. There is usually little or no lag time and the patient should show little to none of their previous symptoms that they experienced during the last infection.

INNATE IMMUNITY

Innate immunity is a rapid non-specific immune response. The innate immune system uses numerous properties such as anatomical barriers, phagocytic cells and important secretory molecules. The first line of defense in innate immunity is the skin (epidermis) which acts as a protective barrier of the internal organs from many infectious agents. Also enzymes such as lysozymes found in tears and saliva can inhibit bacteria growth. Other important components of innate immunity include the presence of phagocytic cells such as neutrophils, eosinophils, macrophages, tissue mast cells, and natural killer (NK) cells; exhibit phagocytic and cytolytic activities; and are important in the inflammatory response and healing. These phagocytic cells also play important roles in activating the adaptive immune response. Other factors that play a role include the activation of the complement system, as well as the production and release of transferrin, interferons and interleukin-1.

COMPLEMENT

Complement is a protein cascade of the **innate immune system** that "complements" the anti-microbial activity of antibodies, hence the name. Complement is made of several small components that activate the main component known as C3. There are three ways in which C3 can be activated. The lectin pathway involves mannan binding lectin, which is capable of binding to carbohydrates of bacteria, leading to C3 activation. The classical pathway occurs through complement recognition of the antibodies (immunoglobulin molecules). The alternative pathway occurs through random activation of C3, which will attack any cells that do not have complement inhibitors, particularly foreign bacteria. Complement is a chemotactic agent for other immune cells, increases immune cell adhesion, increases the permeability of blood vessels, facilitates phagocytosis, aids in transport of immune complexes to areas of phagocytosis, and creates pores in pathogens, which could lead to increased lysis of the cells. Complement also has important roles in B cell stimulation and regulation of the memory response of the immune system.

ADAPTIVE/ANTIBODY-MEDIATED IMMUNITY

Immune host defenses are more specific than innate immune responses and are directed against a specific pathogen or its byproducts. This inducible defense system develops resistance and immunity. **Adaptive/Antibody-mediated (humoral) immunity** begins when a microorganism invades a host and carries antigenic substances, which can be components of the cell wall, structures such as fimbriae, toxins or enzymes. When a macrophage encounters a pathogen, it phagocytizes and destroys it. Then the macrophage displays fragments of the antigen on its surface to activate T cells, which in turn activate B cells, which divide and form plasma cells, which release antibodies that are specific to the antigens. Antibodies are immunoglobulins, of which there are 5 types. The macrophage also forms memory cells, which become part of the permanent immune system. The antibodies bind to antigens, creating what is referred to as the antigen-antibody complex, and destroying the antigen, leading to destruction of the pathogen.

BETA LYMPHOCYTES, T-LYMPHOCYTES, NATURAL KILLER CELLS, AND MACROPHAGES

Beta-lymphocytes (B cells) are developed in the bone marrow and originate from lymphoid stem cells. They make up 15% of white blood cells or lymphocytes that are circulating in the blood at any time. B-cells are important in making antibodies against antigens. **T-lymphocytes (T-Cells)** are cells that eventually give rise to T-cells are formed in the bone marrow from lymphoid stem cells and travel to the thymus, where they mature into T-cells. T-cells are activated in response to an antigen that is presented by an antigen presenting cell. Helper T-cells are important in the stimulation of various lymphocytes, increasing the immune response. Cytotoxic T-cells are important in killing cells that are infected with a certain infectious agent such as a virus. **Natural**

killer cells are formed in the bone marrow from lymphoid cells; natural killer cells are cytotoxic lymphocytes that play a major role in the removal of virally infected cells. They have a role in rejection of tumors as well. **Macrophages** are monocytes that originate from the myeloid stem cells in the bone marrow. Their major function is phagocytosis of infected cells.

Degranulation

Degranulation is a process of the immune system and occurs in mast cells, NK cells, and cytotoxic T cells, as well as other immune cells that involve the release of cytotoxic compounds such as perforin, granzymes, histamine, proteoglycans, and proteases. These compounds are stored in secretory compartments known as granules, and degranulation is the process of their release. These cytotoxic compounds are important in the killing of infected cells and are vital for the immune response.

SCID

SCID stands for **severe combined immunodeficiency disorder**, which is a genetic disorder in which B and T-cells, due to various genetic mutations, are disabled, causing the adaptive immune response to malfunction. Treatment for this disorder originally consisted of living in a self-contained bubble, to keep the patient in a sterile environment away from any pathogens, even normally innocuous diseases, which would be fatal to a patient suffering from this disease. Bone marrow transplant was also a viable treatment; however, this treatment did not show great success until the 1980s. New methods of transplantation, however, have allowed for effective therapy of SCIDs. Recently, new forms of gene therapy have also shown some moderate success in replacing/fixing the genetic defects in the patient that lead to the development of SCIDs.

Common Genetic Mutations

SCID (severe combined immunodeficiency disorder) can be caused by numerous genetic disorders. The moist common mutation occurs in the gamma side chain of the interleukin proteins. The interleukin proteins have essential roles in the development and maturation of B and T cells. If the interleukins are mutated, the B and T cells cannot develop properly. Other causes of SCID include a mutation in the gene that transcribes the protein Janus-kinase-3 which mediates the downstream signaling of the interleukin proteins. Mutations in adenosine deaminase lead to the inhibition of purine breakdown, which has a preventive effect on proliferation and inhibits the immune response by inhibiting lymphocyte proliferation. Also, mutations in the gene's RAG-1 and RAG-2, can lead to an inhibition of V(D)J recombination. V(D)J recombination is the process by which new receptors are made, through recombination of genes, allowing for the diversity of B and T cells to combat the large amount of allergens that insult the body daily.

Immunoglobulins

Immunoglobulins are a class of antibodies and are essential for a functional immune response.

- **IgG**: The most abundant immunoglobulin. It accounts for 75–80% of all antibodies. IgG combats bacterial and viral infections through activation of macrophages and NK cells.
- **IgM**: The largest of the antibodies; first to be produced in response to an infection/antigen. This immunoglobulin accounts for approximately 5 -10% of all antibodies.
- **IgA**: Secreted in tears and saliva. Also found in the digestive, respiratory and urogenital tracts. IgA prevents pathogenic colonization of mucosal membranes. IgA accounts for 10% of all antibodies.

- **IgE**: Found in lungs, skin and mucosal membranes. IgE is essential for allergic reactions, causing the body to react to foreign substances such as food, animal dander, or drugs. Generally in low abundance, IgE is highly elevated in patients with severe allergies, leading to hypersensitivity to normally innocuous allergens.
- **IgD**: Little is known about its function. It's found on immature lymphocytes and may play an important role in the early immune response. IgD accounts for 1% of total immunoglobulin levels.

Monoclonal Antibodies

Monoclonal antibodies are created by using an antigen that is injected, usually multiple times, into an animal. Antibodies (B-cells) form against the antigen. These antibodies are removed from the body and are fused with immortalized cultured myeloma tumor cells that have lost the ability to produce antibodies. This fusion can occur by many means such as electroporation, decreased membrane permeability and recombinant viral infection. This allows for a large number of antibodies to be formed in culture, purified, and used for therapy or for research.

Type I Hypersensitivity

Type I hypersensitivity is considered an immediate hypersensitivity and often leads to an acute allergic or anaphylaxis reaction in people sensitive to a specific antigen. It involves excessive secretion of the IgE immunoglobulin in response to an allergen such as pollen, animal dander, or fungal spores. Symptoms include runny nose, bronchiole constriction, which could lead to restricted breathing and increased asthma. Onset of reaction can occur within seconds or minutes of an antigen challenge. Clinical examples of type I hypersensitivity include allergy induced asthma, allergic conjunctivitis, allergic rhinitis, eczema, and angioedema.

Type II Hypersensitivity

Type II hypersensitivity, also known as cytotoxic hypersensitivity, occurs when IgG immunoglobulins react with antigens on the cell surfaces and develop antibodies against antigens on their own cells. The immunoglobulin/antigen complex can lead to lysis and death of the cell, often damaging tissues of vital organ systems. Onset of reaction can occur within minutes or a few hours after introduction of an antigen. Clinical examples of type II hypersensitivity include Rheumatic Fever, Hashimoto's thyroiditis, Goodpasture's syndrome, autoimmune hemolytic anemia, and pemphigus.

Type III Hypersensitivity

Type III hypersensitivity occurs when a large amount of IgG and IgM form complexes with soluble antigens. This often occurs in response to excess antigens in the blood or decreased levels of antibodies are produced. The immunoglobulin-antigen complexes often are deposited in various tissues such as the skin, kidneys and in the joints. The complexes are removed by the innate complement immune response. Onset can occur within two to six hours after exposure to an antigen. Clinical examples of type III hypersensitivity include systemic lupus erythematosus, Rheumatoid arthritis, serum sickness, subacute bacterial endocarditis, immune-complex glomerulonephritis, or Arthus Reaction.

Type IV Hypersensitivity

Type IV hypersensitivity is also known as delayed hypersensitivity or cell-mediated hypersensitivity. It is known as delayed hypersensitivity because the reaction might take two to three days to occur, while other hypersensitivity reactions are much more rapid. Type IV hypersensitivity is caused when a specific antigen is presented to memory T-cells by an antigen-presenting cell. Memory T-cells can lead to increased presence of inflammatory cells in a particular tissue, inflammation can increase, and tissue damage can occur. In patients sensitive to a specific antigen, the initial induction of inflammation can be observed after a few hours, but the full Type IV hypersensitivity reaction will peak at twenty-four to forty-eight hours. Clinical examples of type IV hypersensitivity include transplant rejection, contact dermatitis, and celiac disease

Hemolytic Disease of the Newborn

Hemolytic disease of the newborn occurs when the mother develops an immune response against the cells of a newborn fetus which leads to an immune attack against the blood cells of the unborn fetus. This type of immune response is known as an alloimmune response. During this reaction, blood cells are broken down which can lead to severe anemia. This can also lead to increased levels of the liver protein bilirubin, which can lead to jaundice, a yellowing of the skin and eyes of the fetus. Anemia can lead to heart failure, respiratory failure, or an enlarged liver, all possibly leading to the death of the fetus before birth or shortly after. This disease can be caused by antigens forming against the A or B antigens on blood. Additionally, antigens that are known as the Rhesus factor (Rh) can lead to a similar response. If a mother is lacking the Rh antigen (Rh-) and has a fetus with an Rh antigen (Rh+), an alloimmune response and hemolytic disease can occur.

Hyposensitivity

Hyposensitivity is when gradual doses of a specific allergen are administered in order to desensitize the patient to the allergic insult and decrease the amount of type I hypersensitivity. This type of immunotherapy shows relative success in decreasing to completely ablating IgE allergic reactions. Direct administration of the allergens into the blood increases IgG levels. As IgG levels increase, it begins to treat allergens as an infectious agent, leading to a cytotoxic response of the immune system, bypassing IgE based hypersensitivity reactions.

Pharmaceutical Sciences

Pharmaceutical Calculations

Units of Measurement

There are two unit measurement systems used in pharmacies. The predominant and standard unit of measurement is the metric system. Some common metric prefixes are mega (million times the base), kilo (thousand times the base), centi (hundred times the base), milli (one thousand of the base), micro (one million of the base), nano (one billion the base), and pico (one trillionth the base). Another system of measurement is the avoirdupois system, which incorporates weight and volume measurements. The weight measurements are grains, scruples, drams, and ounces. The volume measurements are minims, fluidrams, fluid ounces, pints, and quarts.

Units of weight measurement include the following:

- 20 grains = 1 scruple
- 3 scruples = 1 dram
- 8 drams = 1 ounce
- 12 ounces = 1 pound
- Units of volume measure
- 60 minims = 1 fluidram
- 8 fluidrams = 1 fluidounce
- 16 fluidounces = 1 pint
- 2 pints = 1 quart
- 4 quarts = 1 gallon
- Conversion factors
- 1 inch = 2.54 centimeters
- 1 fluidounce = 30 milliliters
- 1 gram = 15.4 grains
- 1 kilogram = 2.20 pounds
- 1 pound = 454 grams
- 1 gallon = 3,785 milliliters

Techniques for Calculating and Converting Dosage

Ratio-proportion is a method that involves cross multiplying of factors and several steps, whereas in dimensional analysis, factors can cancel out, which simplifies the calculation. Some common conversions between units of measurement are as follows:

- 1 pound = 16 ounces = 454 g
- 2.2 pounds = 1 kg
- 3 teaspoons = 1 tablespoon
- 2 T = 1 fluid ounces = 1/8 cup
- 1 cup = 8 fluid ounces
- 1 pint = 16 fluid ounces = 2 cups
- 1 quart = 32 fluid ounces = 4 cups
- 1 gallon = 128 fluid ounces = 16 cups
- 1 teaspoon = 5 mL

- 1 tablespoon = 15 mL
- 1 fluid ounce = 29.6 mL
- 1 cup = 240 mL
- 1 pint = 473 mL
- 1 quart = 946 mL
- 1 gallon = 3,785 mL

Micrograms, Milligrams, Parts per Million, and Parts per Billion

Micrograms are a thousandth the mass of a milligram, which in turn is a thousandth the mass of a gram. Parts per million (ppm) and parts per billion (ppb) are measures of how much of a substance, by mass, is present compared to the solid, in kilograms. Because ppm and ppb are based on kilograms, a substance's amount in milligrams is the same as its amount in ppm, and its amount in micrograms is the same as its amount in ppb.

Determine the number of milligrams of sodium in an infusion of 5 million units of penicillin (2.2 mEq of sodium per million of penicillin, atomic weight of sodium = 23, valence of sodium = 1+).

5 million units × 2.2 mEq = 11,000 moles of cations

Converting Centigrade to Fahrenheit

The conversion of temperatures between Centigrade and Fahrenheit uses the following formula:

$$9\ °C = 5\ °F - 150$$

where C is the temperature in °C and F is the temperature in °F.

For example, a patient's temperature of 101°F in centigrade is calculated via:

°F = 101
9 °C = 5 (101) – 150
9 °C = 355
°C = 39.4°C

Another use is to convert ambient temperature (i.e. room temperature), which is about 25 degrees centigrade, into degrees Fahrenheit. The calculation is:

°C = 25
9 (25) = 5 °F – 150
225 + 150 = 5 °F
375 = 5 °F
°F = 75 °F

Converting Volume to Weight

Conversions between volume and weight involve the specific gravity (SG) or density (D) of the substance. Density is calculated as mass divided by volume. The density of water, the universal solvent, is 1 g/mL or 1 kg/L. The specific gravity is the ratio of a substance's density to that of water. However, if the volume is constant, it can also describe the ratio of a substance's mass or weight to that of water. (Note: Although weight has a slightly different meaning than mass, for Earth's nearly constant gravity, most pharmacists will use mass and weight interchangeably.)

$$SG = \frac{D_{sample}}{D_{H_2O}} \; ; \; Density = \frac{Mass}{Volume}$$

Example

Calculate the weight of a 100 mL mystery solution with a specific gravity of 1.20.

$$SG = 1.2 = \frac{D_{sample}}{1 \text{ g/mL}}$$

D_{sample} = 1.2 g/mL
1.2 g/mL = mass / 100 mL
mass = 120 g

Note that, because specific gravity is defined as the ratio of two similar units, the units go away, leaving specific gravity unitless.

RATES OF ADMINISTRATION

CALCULATING DRIP RATE

Drip rate can be calculated using the following equation:

(Volume × rate) / time = drops per minute

Example: Calculate the drip rate of 100 milliliters of IV fluid that is prescribed to be given over 30 minutes at a rate of 10 drops/mL. The same patient is to receive 1.5 liters of normal saline (IV over four hours). Calculate the rate when 10 drops per milliliter is the rate.

(100 mL × 10 drops/mL) / 30 minutes = 33 drops per minute

(1,500 mL × 10 drops/mL) / 240 minutes = 63 drops per minute

CALCULATING DROPS PER MINUTE

Drops (gtts) per minute can be calculated using the following equation:

(volume × drop factor) / time = drops per minute

Example: A patient must receive 50 milliliters of IV fluid over one hour's time. Calculate the drops per minute when the drop factor is 15. Once this has been administered to the patient, you are required to provide the patient with one liter of 5% dextrose (IV over eight hours). The drop factor is 10. Calculate the number of drops per minute for the 5% dextrose.

(volume × drop factor) / time = corrected rate
(50 mL × 15 drops/mL) / 60 minutes = 25 drops per minute
(volume × drop factor) / time = drops per minute
(1,000 mL × 10) / 480 minutes = 21 drops per minute

Drug Concentrations

Expressing Active Ingredients for Medications

The amount of active ingredient is expressed as the amount per each dosage form, concentration per dosing volume, percent strength (g/mL), ratio strength (active/total), parts per million (mg/L or mcg/g), and parts per billion (mcg/L or ng/g). Ratio strength is another expression of concentration. For example, take a drug formulated as a capsule containing 5% active ingredient. This means that each capsule (or dose) contains 5 parts of the active ingredient per 100 parts of formulated product. The 5% active ingredient can also be expressed as 5:100 or 1:20 (1 part active ingredient per 20 parts of formulated product).

Percentage Weight in Volume

Percentage weight in volume (%w/v) indicates the number of grams per 100 mL of solution.

$$X\%\ {}^{w}/_{v} = \frac{X\text{ g}}{100\text{ mL solution}}$$

Calculate the total %w/v of 50 mL of a 10% w/v tolu balsam solution diluted in an additional 950 mL of water.

$$50\text{mL solution} \times \frac{10\text{g tolu balsam}}{100\text{ mL solution}} = 5\text{g tolu balsam}$$

$$\frac{5\text{ g tolu balsam}}{950\text{ mL} + 50\text{ mL } H_2O} = \frac{5\text{ g}}{1000\text{ mL}}$$

$$\frac{5\text{ g}}{1000\text{ mL}} = \frac{X\text{ g}}{100\text{ mL}}$$

By solving for X, X = 0.5

The new solution is 0.5% w/v

Percentage and Ratio Strengths

The amount of each active ingredient in each dosage form is expressed as a concentration per dosing volume, percentage, ratio strength, or ppm or ppb. Percent is the amount of active ingredient in a total of 100. Percent weight to weight (% w/w) is the number of grams of active ingredient per 100 g of product. Percent weight to volume (% w/v) is the number of grams of active ingredient per 100 mL of product. Percent volume to volume (% v/v) is the number of milliliters of active ingredient per 100 mL of product.

Ratio Strength for 1 Gram Active Ingredient per 1 L of Solution

The following shows 1 g active ingredient per 1L of product solution in mathematical form:

$$\frac{1\text{ g active ingredient}}{1{,}000\text{ mL}} \times \frac{100\text{ mL}}{1\text{ g}} = 0.1\%\ {}^{w}/_{v}\ \text{(or 1: 1,000)}$$

The number of grams required for 10 L of product to ensure it is preserved at a final concentration of active ingredient at 1:10,000.

1:10,000 is 0.0001% active ingredient.

0.0001 g active ingredient in 0.1 L product is 0.0001%, 0.001 g for 1 L, and 0.01 g for 10,000 L.

The amount of grams for 10,000 mL at 0.0001% = 0.1 g

Example of Calculating Ratio Strength

Example: Calculate the ratio strength of 3.5 g of a drug in a 0.15 L solution as a percent and ratio strength. Calculate the same for 3.5 g of a drug in a 0.70 L solution.

The percent strength is found by dividing the amount of drug in grams by the total amount of solution in mL:

$$\frac{3.5\text{ g}}{0.15\text{ L}} \times \frac{1\text{ L}}{1000\text{ mL}} = \frac{3.5\text{ g}}{150\text{ mL}} = 0.023\frac{\text{g}}{\text{mL}} = 2.3\%\text{ w/v}$$

Ratio strength is simply the percentage to 100, 2.3:100 or 23:1000.

For the drug in 0.70 L solution, the percent strength is again found by dividing the amount of drug in grams by the total amount of solution in mL:

$$\frac{3.5\text{ g}}{0.70\text{ L}} \times \frac{1\text{ L}}{1000\text{ mL}} = \frac{3.5\text{ g}}{700\text{ mL}} = 0.005\frac{\text{g}}{\text{mL}} = 0.50\%\text{ w/v}$$

Ratio strength is 5:1000 or 1:200.

Calculating Dose Using Formulas with Parts

Dosing can be calculated using formulas with 'parts.' For instance, consider the following example: Calculate the amount to prepare 100 g of camphorated parachlorophenol, given that camphorated parachlorophenol is 7 parts parachlorophenol to 13 parts camphor.

7 parts parachlorophenol + 13 parts camphor = 20 parts total

$$100\text{ g} \times \frac{7\text{ parts parachlorophenol}}{20\text{ parts total}} = 35\text{ g parachlorophenol}$$

$$100\text{ g} \times \frac{13\text{ parts camphor}}{20\text{ parts total}} = 65\text{ g camphor}$$

Calculating the Constituents of an Active Drug Moiety

When dispensing an **active drug moiety**, information on the constituents of the final drug product must be obtained. These details include the absorbed water, water of hydration, pH, detergents, preservatives, and other items that might affect the consistency of the active drug moiety. The parameters used to calculate the amount of active drug moiety are weight of drug, weight of active drug moiety in the prescription, formula weight of drug complex, fraction dry weight, and formula weight of the active drug moiety in the drug complex.

Weight of drug complex to dispense in grams = (weight of active drug moiety prescribed) × (formula weight of drug complex) / [(fraction dry weight) × (formula weight drug moiety in drug complex)].

Reducing and Enlarging Formulas for Compounding

In order to prepare 25 capsules from a mixture of ketoprofen (2 g), caffeine (3 g), lactose (30 g), and M et div caps (200).

M et div = mix and divide

200 capsules/25 capsules needed = 8/100 = 0.08
ketoprofen (2 g × 0.08 = 0.16 g)
caffeine (3 g × 0.08 = 0.24 g)
lactose (30 g × 0.08 = 2.4 g)

25 capsules require 0.16g ketoprofen, 0.24g caffeine, and 2.4g lactose.

Example of Calculating Weight of Magnesium Chloride to Prepare

Example: Calculate the weight of magnesium chloride required to prepare 100mL of a 0.25M solution and 250mL of a 0.5M solution.

Using a periodic table, the formula weight of magnesium chloride ($MgCl_2$) is calculated to be 95.3g/mol. The molarity of the solution (.25M) must be multipled by the volume required (100mL) and the formula weight of the $MgCl_2$ (95.3g/mol) to find the necessary mass. Don't forget that molarity is in mol/L, so a conversion factor (1L/1000mL) is needed. Thus, for the first solution:

$$\frac{0.25\text{ mol}}{1\text{ L}} \cdot \frac{1\text{ L}}{1000\text{ mL}} \cdot \frac{95.3\text{ g}}{\text{mol}} \cdot 100\text{ mL} = 2.383\text{ g},$$

and for the second solution:

$$\frac{0.5\text{ mol}}{1\text{ L}} \cdot \frac{1\text{ L}}{1000\text{ mL}} \cdot \frac{95.3\text{ g}}{\text{mol}} \cdot 250\ mL = 11.913\ g$$

Example Calculation for Methyldopa

Example: A patient is prescribed methyldopa (25 mg, IV) and flupentixol (5 mg, IM). Assume there are solutions already prepared for them at 50 mg in 5 mL and 40 mg in 2 mL, respectively, and calculate the volume needed to achieve the correct dose for both drugs.

The calculation is as follows for methyldopa:

50 mg / 5 mL = 10 mg/mL concentration of available solution
25 mg / 10 mg /L = 2.5 mL
2.5 mL of the 50 mg per 5 mL solution equals a 25 mg dose

The calculation is as follows for flupentixol:

40 mg / 2 mL = 20 mg/mL concentration of available solution
5 mg / 20 mg/mL = 0.25 mL
0.5 mL of the 40 mg per 2 mL solution equals a 5 mg dose

Example Calculation to Determine Volume Needed for Specific Doses

Example: A patient is prescribed morphine (13 mg, IM) and gentamicin (22 mg, IM). Assume there are solutions already prepared for them at 5 mg in 1 mL and 20 mg in 2 mL, respectively, and calculate the volume needed to achieve the correct dose for both drugs.

The calculation is as follows for **morphine**:

5 mg / 1 mL = 5 mg/mL concentration of available solution
13 mg / 5 mg /mL = 2.6 mL
2.6 mL of the 5 mg per 1 mL solution equals a 13 mg dose

The calculation is as follows for **gentamicin**:

20 mg / 2 mL = 10 mg/mL concentration of available solution
22 mg / 10 mg /mL = 2.2 mL
2.2 mL of the 20 mg per 2 mL solution equals a 22 mg dose

Dose Calculation, Dilution, Concentration, and Alligation

The total dose is calculated by multiplying the number of doses given by the size of the dose. When diluting or concentrating a substance, convert ratio strength to percentage strength. Next, set up a proportion of quantity / concentration = required quantity / required concentration. Stock solutions are generally prepared as a weight to volume (w/v) mixture, and the concentration is expressed as a ratio strength. Alligation is a method of calculating a mixture of products with different percent strengths. Medial and alternate alligation are used. Medial alligation uses the weighted average of percentage strength. Alternate alligation uses the number of parts of a mixture (at least two components).

Alligation Medial

Alligation is the calculation of the weighted average percentage strength of a mixture of at least two substances. Alligation medial is the percent strength (w/w) of alcohol in a mixture and can be calculated with the following:

(Mixture is 1,000 mL 20% (v/v) alcohol + 1,000 mL 60% (v/v) alcohol + 1,000 mL 70% (v/v) alcohol.)

$20 \times 1{,}000 = 20{,}000$
$60 \times 1{,}000 = 60{,}000$
$70 \times 1{,}000 = 70{,}000$

This yields 3,000 @ 150,000 = 150,000/3,000 = 50% (v/v).

Trituration

A trituration is 10% (weight to weight, w/w) of finely powdered or triturated mixtures of a drug. A trituration is the drug in an inert substance. For example, to calculate the weight of colchicine trituration required to prepare 20 doses of 0.20 mg each, one knows that a 10 mg mixture contains 1 mg of colchicine. Next, 10 mg (20 doses × 0.20 mg of drug) / 1 mg drug = 40 mg trituration.

Buffering Solutions and Calculating pH of a Solution

Buffering solutions are used to maintain a specific pH or pH range for a solution. Most buffers are a weak acid or base and a salt of the corresponding acid or base. The pH of a solution can be calculated by using the Henderson-Hasselbalch equation.

- For a weak acid, the pH = pKa + log (salt/acid).
- For a weak base, the pH = pKw – pKb + log (base/salt), where the pKw = 14.

For example, the pH of a solution at 0.15 M in ammonia and 0.025 M in ammonium chloride is as follows: (pKb of ammonia is 4.74)

pH = pKw = pKb + log (base/salt) = 14.00 – 4.74 + log (0.15/0.025) = 8.48

Example of Using Inverse Proportions to Calculate Dilution

Example: You have a 120 mL at 10% stock solution that is diluted to 240 mL final volume. What is the diluted concentration?

Calculate final volume = $\frac{120 \text{ mL}}{240 \text{ mL}} \times 10\% = 5\%$

Calculating Density Factor

The density factor is described as follows:

Density factor = weight of drug / weight of base displaced

Example: Calculate the number of grams of a drug for one suppository medication of 30 mg, density factor of 1.2 (inert ingredient), and weight of suppository at 2.5g.

The calculation for the suppository is as follows:

0.03 g drug / 1.2 = 0.025 g inert ingredient
2.5 g – 0.025 g = 2.475 g inert per suppository
0.025 g drug

Calculating Volume of Correct Dose in a Syringe

Example: An oral dose of 600 mg is required of a medication at a concentration of 200 mg/5 cc. Calculate the volume to equal the correct dose.

Since 1 cc is 1 mL, the concentration of the medication is 200 mg / 5 mL = 40 mg/mL. The volume is 15 mL = 600 mg / 40 mg/mL. The 15 mL dose can be administered correctly by identifying the leading and trailing ring of the plunger of the syringe. The leading ring is the tip of the plunger closest to the needle, while the trailing ring is farthest from the needle. Another important aspect to using the correct syringe is to choose one that is calibrated in milliliters instead of milligrams.

Calculating Dose When Converting from PO to IM

Example: A patient's psychiatrist wants to change the drug therapy from 20 mg PO bid of haloperidol to haloperidol decanoate. Calculate the dose of haloperidol decanoate.

Haloperidol and **haloperidol decanoate** are drug therapy options for schizophrenia. The dose range is 1–100 mg/day (PO) and 50–300 mg IM (once every four weeks), respectively. A patient's psychiatrist wants to change the drug therapy from 20 mg PO bid of haloperidol to haloperidol decanoate. To calculate the injection dose, which is equivalent to the current oral dose, one should multiple by a factor of 10. Therefore, 20 mg bid × 10 = 200 mg IM. There are four main drug therapies for schizophrenia including chlorpromazine (Thorazine), thioridazine (Mellaril), fluphenazine (Prolixin), and haloperidol (Haldol). The dosage range for these drugs is 50–2,000 mg/day, 50–800 mg/day, 1–65 mg/day (PO) or 12.5–75 mg IM every two weeks, and 1–100 mg/day (PO) or 50–300 mg IM every four weeks, respectively.

Ionization and pH-Partition Theory

The absorption of a drug can be defined by the pH-partition theory. This theory states that drugs are absorbed by passive diffusion through biological membranes. The amount of absorption depends on the fraction of the un-ionized form of the drug and the pH of the biological fluids near the membrane. The degree of ionization depends on the a*cid dissociation constant* (pKa) and the pH. The pKa of a drug can be described as a strong acid (< 2), weak acid (2–7), weak base (7–10), or strong base (>10). The dissociation constant is important because it describes the dissociation into a conjugate base and proton or a conjugate acid and hydroxide ion. When drugs are formulated for oral delivery, the gastrointestinal epithelia act as a lipophilic barrier to ionized drugs. However, un-ionized drugs are more hydrophilic and are absorbed more easily.

Osmolality and Osmolarity

Molarity and Molality

A solution is made from some amount of solute dissolved into a solvent (usually water). Molarity and molality both describe how much solute is present in a given solution, but they are calculated from slightly different quantities. **Molarity** is the measure of **moles** of **solute** per **liter (volume)** of **solution**, measured in units of molar [M], or mol/L. **Molality** is the measure of **moles** of **solute** per **kilogram (mass)** of **solvent**, measured in units of molal [m], or more commonly mol/kg.

In water, which has a density of 1 kg/L or 1 g/mL, molarity and molality are basically equivalent. For solvents whose densities are not close to 1, like alcohol (.789g/mL) and diethyl ether (0.713g/mL), molarity and molality will differ significantly.

Electrolytes, Cations, Anions, Osmolarity, and Osmolality

Electrolytes dissociate in solution into ions. Examples are NaCl, KCl, MgCl2, and MgSO4. Nonelectrolytes do not dissociate when in solution. Examples are dextrose and urea. **Cations** and **anions** are ions in solution that move toward the opposite charge. Cations are positively charged, whereas anions are negatively charged. The cathode (negative electrode) is where the cations migrate, and the anode (positive electrode) is where the anions migrate. **Osmolarity** is the number of millimoles of solute per liter of solution, and **osmolality** is the number of moles of solute per kilogram of solvent. Osmolarity is not equivalent to osmolality.

Osmoles

Osmoles differ from moles in that osmoles are concerned with **dissociated ions**. Electrolytic solutes will dissociate into their component ions when placed in a polar solvent such as water, resulting in the number of moles of dissolved ion particles (osmoles) being some multiple of the number of moles of solute. For example, the electrolyte NaCl will dissociate into one sodium ion and one chlorine ion, so one mole of NaCl placed in a polar solvent would contribute two osmoles.

Osmolarity and osmolality have essentially the same distinction as molarity and molality. **Osmolarity** is measured as osmoles per liter of **solution** (Osm/L) while **osmolality** is measured as osmoles per kg of **solvent** (Osm/kg). In water, which has a density of 1 kg/L or 1 g/mL, osmolarity and osmolality are basically equivalent. For solutes that do not dissociate in solution, osmolarity and osmolality are redundant, since they would be equivalent to molarity and molality, respectively.

Millimoles and Milliosmoles

Moles signify the amount of a substance, given as 6.022×10^{23} atoms or molecules. Osmoles signify the number of moles of a solute which contributes to osmolarity. This information is often used when dispensing or compounding electrolytes and other nutrients.

The molar concentration of a 5% w/v $MgCl_2$ solution is calculated as follows:

$$\frac{1 \text{ mol } MgCl_2}{95 \text{ g } MgCl_2} \times \frac{5 \text{ g } MgCl_2}{100 \text{ mL } H_2O} \times \frac{1{,}000 \text{ mL}}{1 \text{ L}} = 0.53 \frac{\text{mol } MgCl_2}{\text{L } H_2O} = 0.53 \text{ M of } MgCl_2 \text{ in } H_2O$$

That is, 5% w/v $MgCl_2$ solution signifies a solution of 5 grams of $MgCl_2$ in 100 mL water. The mass of the $MgCl_2$ is converted into moles and the volume of water is converted to liters to give the molarity.

The osmolar concentration of the same 5% w/v $MgCl_2$ solution is calculated as follows:

$$\frac{1\text{ mol MgCl}_2}{95\text{ g MgCl}_2} \times \frac{5\text{ g MgCl}_2}{100\text{ mL H}_2\text{O}} \times \frac{1{,}000\text{ mL}}{1\text{ L}} \times \frac{3\text{ mol ions}}{1\text{ mol MgCl}_2} = 1.58\frac{\text{mol ions}}{\text{L H}_2\text{O}}$$
$$= 1.58\text{ Osm/L of MgCl}_2\text{ in H}_2\text{O}$$

As each mole of $MgCl_2$ will ionize into two Cl ions and one Mg ion, its solution has 3x as many osmoles as moles.

Equivalent Weight

The equivalent weight, in terms of charge, represents the mass of a substance that is needed to produce one mole of its charge. Therefore, an equivalent is the molecular weight of an ion divided by its valence. For monovalent ions (ions with only one equivalent charge) like Cl^-, Na^+, or NO_3^-, this will be equal to the ion's molecular weight (here 35.5 eq, 23 eq, and 62 eq). For ions with multiple charges, it will be different; e.g., Mg^{2+} is 12.2 eq, SO_4^{2-} is 48 eq, and PO_4^{3-} is 31.7 eq.

Osmoles describe the total number of charges of a solution. This usually includes both cations and anions, whereas the equivalent weights of simple substances usually only include one charge or the other.

Like other units, equivalents and osmoles may use SI prefixes and specify smaller units like milliequivalents (meq) or microosmoles (μOsm).

Isotonicity

Prescriptions of parenteral formulations of medications must be accurately calculated in order to prevent tissue damage and possible death. A net osmolarity difference results in a pressure difference across a semipermeable membrane (e.g. a cell membrane) because of the diffusion of solvent or solute. Parenteral medications must use similar osmolalities to those of the patient's cells, or risk increased and intolerable pressures across these delicate membranes.

In terms of semipermeable membranes like cell membranes, the net osmolarity refers to the difference in concentration of a specific solute between the two sides of the membrane. The net tonicity refers to the total osmotic pressure difference from all solutes between the two sides of the membrane. In this way (compared to a neutral cell), you can have an iso-osmotic solution which is not isotonic, or vice versa. A normal cell is usually taken to be approximately both isotonic and iso-osmotic to a 5% dextrose/0.9% saline solution. The isotonic reference standard is plasma (280–300 mOsm/L), and the tonicity of a solution can be calculated by using the dissociation constant of the particles.

Electrolyte Solutions and Calculations

Electrolytes are vital for optimal health, and patients who do not have the optimal level of electrolytes may benefit from electrolyte therapy. Millimoles are calculated with the moles (measurement of the amount of substance), atomic weight, molecular weight (sum of all atomic weights), and molar solution (1 mole of solute in 1 L). For example, the molar concentration of a 10% $MgCl_2$ solution is calculated as follows:

5% = 5 g $MgCl_2$ / 100 mL
MW of $MgCl_2$ = 95
1 mole $MgCl_2$ / 95 g $MgCl_2$ = 5 g $MgCl_2$ / 100 mL = 1,000 mL / 1 L = 1.10

Since electrolytes are often prescribed in equivalents and not in mass, it is important to calculate them. An electrolyte is an ion. An equivalent for an ion is the amount required to replace or react with 1 mole of hydrogen. Monovalent ions have an equivalent of 1 Eq/mole. It is important to note that millimoles of a substance do not necessarily equal milliequivalents.

Dissociating Solute

The correct osmolality of a solution must be calculated prior to prescription and dispensing. When several solutions are combined, one must know the dissociation of each component in order to calculate the tonicity of the entire solution. The dissociation factor (i) is the ratio of the total number of particles after dissociation to the number of molecules before dissociation. Typically, it is assumed that the solute will dissociate into two parts, but not all do. For example, the dissociation factor of a solute that dissociates 60% in solution into two ions is

$i = [(100-60) + 60 \times 2] / 100 = 1.6$

However, if the solute dissociated 40% in solution into three ions, its dissociation factor would be

$i = [(100-40) + 40 \times 3] / 100 = 1.8$

These factors for strong electrolytes can be estimated as the number of ions they dissociated into, and even the percentage that dissociates may vary by concentration.

Dissociation Factors of Magnesium Chloride

Magnesium chloride ($MgCl_2$) is an electrolyte with three ions (Mg, Cl, and Cl). This electrolyte typically dissociates at 80%. Thus

$i = [(100-80) + 80 \times 3] / 100 = 2.6$

Sodium chloride (NaCl) typically dissociates at 80%, as well, but has only two ions. Thus

$i = [(100-80) + 80 \times 2] / 100 = 1.8$

Sugars like dextrose don't dissociate in solution, so

$i = [(100-0) + 0 \times 1] / 100 = 1.0$

Sodium Chloride Equivalent

The tonicity of a solution is calculated by summing the **sodium chloride equivalents** of each drug in solution. The sodium chloride equivalent (E) is the number of grams of sodium chloride that yields the same tonicity as 1 g of the drug. It can be calculated as follows:

$$E = \frac{Molar\ weight\ of\ NaCl \cdot Drug\ dissociation\ factor}{Molar\ weight\ of\ drug \cdot NaCl\ dissociation\ factor}$$

Here, the Molar weight of NaCl is 58.5 g/mol, the NaCl dissociation factor is 1.8, and the Drug dissociation factor is characterized by the variable *i*, as discussed earlier. Plugging in these values, the formula is simplified to:

$$E = \frac{58.5 \cdot i}{1.8 \cdot MW_{drug}}$$

Henderson-Hasselbalch Equation

The Henderson-Hasselbalch equation states that the pH of a drug in solution is equal to its acid dissociation constant (pKa) plus the logarithm of the concentration of the drug's acidic form divided by the concentration of the drug's basic form.

$$\mathrm{pH} = \mathrm{pKa} + \log\frac{[A^-]}{[HA]}$$

Thus, the pH of a drug will equal the pKa when the ionized drug is at the same concentration as the unionized drug:

$$If\ pH = pKa, \log\frac{[A^-]}{[HA]} = \log\frac{[Ionized\ drug]}{[Unionized\ drug]} = 0,$$

$$\frac{[Ionized\ drug]}{[Unionized\ drug]} = 10^0 = 1, and$$

$$necessarily\ [Ionized\ drug] = [Unionized\ drug]$$

This will happen when the salt/acid ratio equals 1; this unique situation is known as the half-neutralization point. In addition, the half-neutralization point is the pH where a buffer has its optimal buffering capacity. An optimal buffering capacity maintains the drug in solution, along with the other excipients of the formulation, and allows for accurate dispensing of the required dosage.

Nutritional Needs

Parenteral Nutrition

Parenteral nutrition is for patients who cannot consume food and process its components with the gastrointestinal tract. Parenteral nutrition is provided for patients with severe acute pancreatitis, short bowel syndrome, and Crohn's disease. Parenteral nutrition contains protein, fat, dextrose, sodium, potassium, calcium, phosphate, magnesium, multivitamins, and trace elements. One drawback to parenteral nutrition is metabolic, where hyperglycemia, hypokalemia, hypophosphatemia, hypomagnesemia, and hyponatremia may occur. Other complications are acid-base and trace-element disorders, fatty acid deficiency, hepatic steatosis, anatomical problems, and infections. The anatomical problems associated with parenteral nutrition are pneumothorax or subclavian artery injury or deep vein thrombosis. Infections can occur around the catheter when the environment is not sterile.

Monitoring

There are several laboratory tests that should be performed to assess the patient's nutritional level. The first test is for electrolytes (potassium, sodium, chloride, calcium, magnesium, and phosphate). The next tests are for serum glucose and bicarbonate. Other tests are for body weight of the patient to track weight excess, which could indicate fluid overload or fat deposition if greater than 0.5 lb/day. Other tests are for proteins (albumin, prealbumin, and transferrin) and serum creatinine. Liver function test (aspartate aminotransferase, alanine aminotransferase, alkaline phosphate, lactate dehydrogenase, and bilirubin. Serum triglycerides should be measured before the first dose of parenteral nutrition and weekly thereafter.

Total Parenteral Nutrition (TPN)

Total parenteral nutrition (TPN) calculates the amount of electrolytes, calories, essential fatty acids, vitamins, and fluids necessary for proper nutrition. TPN is often expressed in milliequivalents (mEq). For example, calculate the number of calories present in the following solution:

Nutrient at 5.0 kcal of energy per gram
4% nutrient (in solution)
200 ml (volume of stock solution)
200 ml × (4 g nutrient/100 ml) × 5.0 kcal/g = 40 kcal

Purpose and Types

Total parenteral nutrition (TPN) is a diet formulated solely for intravenous, subcutaneous, or other nonalimentary administration. TPN is required by patients who are not able to eat on their own or who are not able to get enough nutritional requirements from what they do consume. The diet combines protein, carbohydrate, fat, vitamin, and mineral constituents. This combination provides the patient with adequate amino acids, monosaccharides, and electrolytes. Patients who are unable to consume food (Crohn's disease, inflammatory bowel, and late-stage cancers) benefit from the TPN diet.

Nutritional Support for Patients with Respiratory Failure

Parenteral nutrition for patients with respiratory failure incorporates a lipid formulation of 4.25% amino acid, 15% dextrose, and 40% to 50% lipids. EN formulations have 40% to 50% lipids, while Oxepa is a low-carbohydrate enteral formulation that has antioxidants and additional fatty acids, which help to reduce inflammation responses in damaged cells. Consequently, the risk of exacerbating the respiratory symptoms with weight gain or increased inflammation may be avoided. Weight gain in patients with respiratory failure can result in respiratory acidosis due to increased carbon dioxide production.

Enteral Nutrition

Enteral nutrition (EN) is necessary for patients who are unable or refuse to eat, even though they are capable of consuming food and breaking it down. There are several indications for EN use, including cardiac failure, hepatic failure, gastrointestinal failure, neurological impairment, and cancer/HIV. The apparatuses used for EN are either a gastrostomy (either a G-tube or a percutaneous endoscopic gastrostomy), jejunostomy, or through nasal tube feeding, the latter being for short-term EN. Complications that arise from EN are aspiration pneumonia, diarrhea, constipation, nasal or esophageal injury, hyperglycemia, hypokalemia, and hypophosphatemia.

Malnutrition

Malnutrition is undernutrition or obesity. Protein undernutrition is caused by decreased intake of nutrients (starvation) or a change in metabolism (trauma or infection). Obesity is another form of malnutrition and involves higher-than-normal caloric intake, particularly of carbohydrate and fats, change in metabolism (genetic predisposition), or through a sedentary lifestyle. Dietary reference intakes (DRIs) are recommended amounts of particular nutrients needed to maintain a healthy diet. The DRI for fiber is recommended at 20–35 g per day. The DRI for calcium is at 1,200–1,500 mg per day (adolescents) and 1,000 mg per day (adult men younger than 65 years and adult women older than 50 years). Multivitamins are important for achieving the recommended DRIs, particularly for pregnant and lactating women, the elderly, vegetarians, and those consuming a diet low in calories.

Marasmus, Kwashiorkor, and Obesity

Marasmus and kwashiorkor are both types of malnutrition. Marasmus is indicative of very low stores of fat and muscle but with normal biochemical and immune measurements. Kwashiorkor is described as having a normal store of fat and muscle, but with low biochemical and immunological measurements. Obesity is another type of malnutrition where the body weight is 120% or greater of ideal body weight. Another indicator of obesity is BMI. There are three classes of obesity by BMI: class I (BMI is 30–35), class II (BMI is 35–40), and class III (BMI is >40).

Components of a Nutritional Assessment

The components of nutritional assessment are history and physical examination, anthropometrics, biochemical assessment, and immune assessment. The history and nutritional assessment involves a determination of dietary intake (anorexia, hyperphagia, and taste alterations), pathology (cancer or burns), effects on organs (diarrhea and constipation), appearance (edema and cachexia), skin (scaling or decubitus ulcers), musculoskeletal (decrease in muscle mass and slower growth), neurological (lower sensory ability and encephalopathy), and hepatic (jaundice and hepatomegaly). The next factor is anthropometrics, which is body fat measurement. The biochemical assessment involves laboratory tests for serum albumin, prealbumin, and creatinine. The immune assessment involves laboratory tests to determine the total lymphocyte count, cell-mediated immunity, and skin tests to common antigens.

Calculating Caloric Requirements for Daily Nutrition

Daily nutrition is composed of total calories (carbohydrate, fat, and protein). The following are the recommendations:

- 25 kcal/kg/day (normal)
- 30 kcal/kg/day (infection or trauma)
- 35 kcal/kg/day (head injury)
- 40 kcal/kg/day (burns over greater than 50% of the body)

The major nutrients are glucose, fat, and protein. Per gram of metabolism, glucose (carbohydrate) is worth 3.4 kcal, fat is worth 9 kcal, and protein is worth 4 kcal. For normal patients, the suggested intake of protein per day is 0.8 g/kg, while 2 g/kg is recommended for patients with head injury. One method to calculate kcal needed by a patient is to multiply the basal energy expenditure (BEE) by the stress factor to determine the kcal required per day. The stress level is 1, 1.3, 1.5, and 2 for normal, infection, major trauma, and severe burns, respectively.

Additional Essential Nutrients

There are several nutrients required for a healthy diet. These include water, electrolytes (sodium, chloride, potassium, calcium, phosphorus, and magnesium), vitamins, and trace elements. The amount of water recommended each day is 35 mL/kg/day. For example, a healthy 35-year-old female at 66 inches and a normal BMI would need to consume 2.065 L of water per day.

Electrolytes

The other nutrients are electrolytes and are listed below for adults:

- Sodium (60–100 mEq/day), Chloride (60–100 mEq/day)
- Potassium (60–100 mEq/day), Calcium (5–15 mEq/day)
- Phosphorus (20–45 mmol/day), Magnesium (10–20 mEq/day)

Vitamins

Vitamins are also a source of nutrients, and 12 or 13 vitamins are typically included in each dose. The recommended intake of vitamins (per day) is listed below:

- A: 3,300 IU
- D: 200 IU
- E: 10 IU
- K: 150 IU
- B1: 6 mg
- B2: 3.6 mg
- B5: 6 mg
- B7: 60 mcg
- B9: 600 mcg
- B12: 5 mcg

Trace Elements

The final type of nutrient is trace elements like zinc (3–5 mg/day), copper (0.5–1.2 mg/day), chromium (10–15 mcg/day), manganese (50–100 mcg/day), and selenium (40–80 mcg/day).

Nutritional Assessment in Patients with Crohn's Disease

Skinfold measurements of the triceps, biceps, subscapular, and suprailiac muscles are often performed to assess nutritional health in patients with Crohn's disease and other diseases. Measurements of less than the fifth percentile may indicate a nutritional deprivation. These patients may require additional caloric intake in order to receive enough protein, fatty acids, vitamins, and trace minerals.

Nutritional Needs for Patients with Critical Burn Injuries

Hyperglycemia is commonly diagnosed in critically ill patients (intensive care), and administration of insulin during this critical care time frame helps maintain the blood glucose between 80–110 mg/dL. Maximum blood glucose of 110 mg/dL rather than 200 mg/dL is recommended for critical care patients. Due to the administration of insulin, resistance may be observed. Burn patients typically have a higher daily caloric need (2.0–2.5g/kg/day). In addition, it is difficult to determine the patient's nitrogen needs due to the loss of tissue. The estimated caloric requirement for burn patients is dependent on the amount of body surface area (BSA) burned, and is as follows:

$$\text{Requirement } in\ kcal = \text{BSA} + 25 \cdot \%\text{BSA burned}$$

Medicinal Chemistry

Biologic Principal of ADME

ADME stands for absorption, distribution, metabolism and excretion. How a drug is absorbed by the body, is related to the site of absorption and related to physiochemical aspects of the drug. The fraction of the drug absorbed is called fa. It is important to remember that only the fraction of the drug unbound to protein fup, causes a pharmacological effect in the body. Distribution of a drug is related to how much of the drug is unbound to protein and how much of the drug is unbound to tissue fut. Fifty percent of all drugs undergo hepatic metabolism via P450 CYP enzymes. The amount of drug that does not undergo hepatic metabolism is the amount of drug that is available for pharmacological effect. Most drugs are primarily excreted through the kidneys and into urine. Some drugs are also excreted unchanged in fecal matter. Monitoring of renal function is vital for drugs that are excreted renally as compromised renal function may hinder drug excretion and cause unwanted adverse events.

Methylene Shuffle

Absorption, solubility and permeability of a compound can be altered in response to the polarity of the compound. In drug designing, the polarity of the compound must be altered in order to achieve a drug that has better absorption, solubility and permeability. **Methylene shuffle** is a technique used to alter the hydrophobic characteristics of a drug compound by substituting large alkyl groups of a compound with smaller groups, which causes the polarity of the compound to increase. This will cause the drug to have greater absorption and reach the therapeutic target with greater efficiency.

Drug Distribution

Distribution is the movement of a drug through the bloodstream to the site of action. Factors that affect distribution include:

- **Blood flow**: Areas with no blood flow (abscess) or limited blood flow (tumor) may impede distribution.
- **Ability to exit bloodstream**: In most capillary beds, drugs are able to pass through pores into the tissues, but capillaries in the brain-blood barrier have pores that are too small, so water-soluble drugs cannot pass through this barrier although lipid-soluble drugs and some with a transport system can pass through the capillary cells rather than pores. Additionally, CNS capillaries contain P-glycoprotein, a transporter that pumps drugs out of the cells and back into the peripheral bloodstream. At birth, the blood-brain barrier is not fully developed yet, so some drugs may pass through. A partial placental barrier also protects the fetus, but lipid-soluble drugs readily pass to the fetus. Drugs that bind to serum proteins, such as albumin, are unable to leave the bloodstream because albumin molecules are too large. Volume of distribution (IV drug dose divided by plasma concentration) determines the rate at which an IV drug passes into tissue.
- **Ability to enter cells**: This may vary according to solubility and the presence of a transport system.

Drug Metabolism

Drug metabolism involves biotransformation (structure of drugs altered by enzymes). Most metabolic actions occur in the liver through hepatic microsomal enzymes (P450 enzyme system) with three enzyme families, designated as CYP1, CYP2 and CYP3. These enzymes catalyze reactions using drugs as substrates. Drug metabolism may result in accelerated excretion of the drug (converts lipid-soluble drugs into water-soluble), inactivation (converts active to inactive compounds), increased therapeutic action (such as conversion of codeine into morphine), activation of "prodrugs" (an inactive compound becomes active), increased toxicity (safe compound converts to toxic) or decreased toxicity (toxic compound converts to safe). The rate of metabolism may be affected by numerous factors:

- **Age**: Liver unable to adequately metabolize drugs until after age one, and liver disease may impair drug metabolism.
- **Induction**: Some drugs cause increased synthesis of drug-metabolizing enzymes (induction), increasing the rate of metabolism of that drug and other drugs as well.
- **First-pass**: Some drugs are rapidly inactivated during the first pass through the liver if administered orally, so different forms of administration may be necessary.

- **Nutrition**: Co-factors necessary for metabolism may be missing with poor nutrition.
- **Drug-drug interactions**: Competition may decrease metabolism of one or both drugs.

Chemical Reaction Phases of Drug Metabolism

Drug metabolism includes two chemical reaction phases that convert one form of a chemical to another:

- **Functionalization (Phase I) reactions** in which functional groups on the drugs are exposed to increase polarity include:
  - *Oxidative*: Xenobiotics (foreign substances) undergo oxidation by Cytochrome 450 enzymes and other enzymes, such as monoamine oxidases and xanthine oxidase, in first pass sites, primarily the liver, in order to make the substances more hydrophilic. A polar functional group (ex. -OH) is introduced during this process.
  - *Reductive*: Reduction results in production of polar functional groups (ex. amino, hydroxyl) in some drug molecules, such as those containing nitrogen, carbonyl, and halogens.
  - *Hydrolytic*: A substantive chemical change occurs in esters and amides with esters forming carboxylic acids and alcohols. Prodrugs are converted during hydrolysis to active metabolites.
- **Biotransformation (Phase II) reactions**: Conjugation reactions occur primarily in products of phase I reactions and are catalyzed by transferase enzymes. Reactive metabolites that cause adverse reactions are formed during this stage

Drug Excretion

Excretion of most drugs is through the kidneys, with water-soluble compounds excreted more readily than lipid-soluble compounds, although the intestines (drugs released by the liver in bile and excreted through the intestines) and the liver (through biotransformation of drugs) also have a role. Renal excretion functions include:

- **Glomerular filtration**: Fluid and small molecules are filtered into the urine. Glomerular filtration prevents large molecules, such as blood cells and drugs bound to large proteins, from passing through.
- **Passive tubular reabsorption**: Lipid-soluble drugs are reabsorbed into the bloodstream.
- **Active tubular secretion**: Pump drugs from the blood into the urine.

Elimination half-time is the time needed to reduce plasma concentrations to 50% during elimination. Usually the equivalent of 5 half-times is needed to completely eliminate a drug. Five half-times are also needed to achieve steady-state plasma concentrations if giving doses intermittently. Context-sensitive half-time, in contrast, is the time needed to reach a specific amount of decrease (50%, 60%) after stopping administration of a drug.

Enthalpy and Entropy

Enthalpy is defined with the equation **H = U + PV.** H = enthalpy, U =internal energy of the system, P= pressure, and V= volume. Enthalpy is an important calculation to determine the energy costs of bringing atoms together, such as developing a drug compound. **Entropy** is the tendency of all energy to go toward an inert state. Entropy is the tendency of all molecules and compounds through spontaneous changes to eventually fall into the lowest energy state of the system.

Energy Minimization

States of lower energy are generally more stable and based on the laws of thermodynamics and entropy; molecules will eventually adopt these lower energy states. The concept of **energy minimization** is to design or alter the geometric design of a drug compound to reduce its energy state, thus increasing the compounds stability. If a drug compound is not at the lowest possible energy state, often times a new geometric configuration would be adopted, decreasing the stability of the drug, decreasing the efficacy, and possibly increasing unwanted toxicity.

Molecular Docking

Molecular docking is computational technique to study the interaction of two or more molecules. This technique is often used to model binding of drug compounds to various receptors and other possible therapeutic targets. This method is an important technique in rational drug design. There are generally two techniques that are commonly used in molecular docking including shape complementation and simulation. Shape complementation models how a ligand can interact with the active region receptor based on geometric shape. This can be used to create a drug compound that is complementary in shape to the receptor. The simulation technique is more complicated, but models what is observed biologically. A ligand is separated by a distance from the enzyme and the ligand is allowed to move until it finds the best fit. This method calculates total energy that is expended in response to the ligand binding at different orientations. This method allows for design of a drug at the lowest possible energy state.

Pharmacophore

A pharmacophore is the active ingredient of a drug that is necessary for the biological effect of the compound. Pharmacophores are often a geometric moiety of a molecule. Molecules with similar pharmacophores will often have similar biological effects, although absorption, distribution, metabolism and excretion of similar molecules may differ greatly. A large part of drug development is spent looking for (molecular mining) and developing new pharmacophores for already existing drugs, in hopes of finding a compound that has greater efficacy against a certain disease state, but show less chance of toxicity.

Lead Compound

A lead compound is an important component of drug development. It is generally the initial compound that is discovered by high throughput screening that inhibits a specific biological/therapeutic target. The lead compound is generally the starting point for other drugs, whose structure can be altered in the drug development process, providing compounds with optimal absorption, distribution, metabolism and excretion as well as efficacy, in hopes of eventually marketing the compound as a treatment against a desired disease state.

QSAR

The **quantitative structure-activity relationship (QSAR)** is a mathematical and statistical model that quantitatively measures a correlative relationship between the pharmacological activity and structure of compounds, which are studied and measured for possible therapeutic drug development. The basic hypothesis is that similarly structured molecules will have similar pharmacological effects; however, slight changes between each compound may alter the activity of the compound including different absorption, different excretion rate, different biotransformation, and different activity levels. Often QSAR is used to find more effective and safe alternative drugs for already marketed therapies.

Lipinski's Rule of Five

Christopher **Lipinski proposed five sets of rules** in order to predict the permeability and absorption of a given compound and determine if the drug is a likely candidate to be absorbed via oral administration. The rules use cut-off values before the compound is considered likely to be absorbed readily by mouth. These rules include that the compound must have less than or equal to five hydrogen bonds, the log P value (partition coefficient) of the compound must be less than five, the compound must not have a molecular weight over 500 daltons, and the compound must have hydrogen bond acceptors (electronegative atoms) that are less than or equal to ten. These rules do not tell if a compound can be used as an effective drug. Other model tests will need to be performed such as QSAR.

Pharmacology and Toxicology

Broad-Spectrum Antibiotics and Narrow-Spectrum Antibiotics

Broad-spectrum antibiotics are a type of antibiotics that generally used in fighting a large range of bacterial infections and can be effective against both gram-negative and gram-positive bacteria. Narrow spectrum antibiotics, however, are more specific, generally effective against a certain type or class of bacteria. Broad spectrum antibiotics are often used as an initial line of defense against an infection, particularly when little is known about the bacteria that caused this infection. Antibiotic stewardship is encouraged whenever broad spectrum antibiotics are administered, with constant reassessment for opportunities to narrow or de-escalate. Also, these types of antibiotics are used when bacteria have become resistant to more specific therapies or when infections involve multiple types of bacteria. Augmentin is an example of a broad-spectrum antibiotic. **Narrow-spectrum antibiotics** such as metronidazole are used when more is known about the underlying infection.

Mechanism of Actions of the Carbapenem Class of Antibiotics

Carbapenems belong to the beta-lactam class of antibiotics. Carbapenems are broad-spectrum antibiotics that include imipenem/cilastatin, meropenem and ertapenem. Carbapenem are effective against many types of bacteria, by inhibiting peptidoglycan synthesis of the cell wall. These compounds are highly resistant to the bacterial enzyme known as beta-lactamase. Beta-lactamase generally can inhibit the activity of beta-lactam antibiotics, by breaking the bonds of the ring structure known as beta-lactam nuclease of the antibiotic molecule.

Mechanism of Actions of the Metronidazole Class of Antibiotics

Metronidazole is an antibiotic that is converted, in anaerobic bacteria, into the active drug, which inhibits and disrupts the double helix structure of DNA, inhibiting DNA synthesis and translation of DNA into mRNA. Metronidazole can be used to combat bacterial infections of various anaerobes including *Entamoeba histolytica*. Adverse reactions include nausea; allergic reactions; and thrombophlebitis, inflammation of veins due to a blood clot. Alcohol is contraindicated with this class of antibiotics; it can lead to nausea, dizziness and tachycardia (very rapid beating of the heart).

Penicillins

Penicillins are a class of β-lactam antibiotics, named in response to the β-lactam ring found in the chemical structure of these antibiotic compounds. Penicillins bind important proteins in the bacterial cell wall, known as penicillin binding proteins (PBPs), inhibiting the synthesis of the cell wall, leading to lysis of the bacteria. There is a large variety of classes of penicillins including natural penicillins (Penicillin G, penicillin V), penicillinase-resistant penicillins (oxacillin, nafcillin, cloxacillin, dicloxacillin), and aminopenicillins, carboxypenicillins (carbenicillin, ticarcillin), and ureidopenicillins (piperacillin). Additionally, β-lactamase inhibitors (clavulanic acid, sulbactam, and tazobactam) are used with penicillins to treat resistant bacteria. These drugs have a wide range of activity against different bacterial species. Adverse reactions include severe allergy, nausea, seizures, hypokalemia, hyponatremia, cholestatic jaundice, and hemolytic anemia.

Aminoglycosides

Aminoglycosides are a class of antibiotics, which include such antibiotics as neomycin, kanamycin, tobramycin and gentamicin. By binding to a ribosomal subunit (30S) during translation, aminoglycosides can inhibit the protein synthesis of the bacteria. Aminoglycosides generally are used against gram-negative bacteria such as *E.coli*, *Klebsiella*, and *Pseudomonas*, but can be used against certain gram positive bacteria as well, such as *Enterococcus* when combined with penicillin or vancomycin. These patients should be monitored for potential side effects including reversible kidney damage and irreversible damage to the important structures of the ear, leading to vertigo and possible hearing loss. These antibiotics are also used if the patient has acquired a gram-negative bacterial infection that is severe, resistant to other treatment, or when broad coverage is needed.

Topoisomerase Inhibitors Agents

Topoisomerase inhibitors are used as anti-neoplastic therapies. There are two classes of inhibitors that either inhibits topoisomerase I or topoisomerase II. Topoisomerase enzymes have important regulatory roles in DNA replication and transcription. They can regulate the supercoiled structure of chromosomes by nicking the strands at either one strand of DNA (topoisomerase I) or both strands of DNA (topoisomerase II), helping stabilize the DNA-enzyme complex, leading to proper replication and transcription to occur. Inhibitors of these enzymes can retard growth, retard transcription and can lead to increased apoptosis of cancer cells. Commonly used topoisomerase I inhibitors used as anti-neoplastic agents include irinotecan and topotecan. Commonly used topoisomerase II inhibitors used as anti-neoplastic drugs include doxorubicin, daunorubicin, epirubicin, mitoxantrone, and etoposide.

Mechanism of Action of Alkylating Agents

Alkylating agents are used as anti-cancer drugs. They act by altering the structure of DNA, which inhibits DNA synthesis as well as transcription. The drugs can covalently link to nucleotides causing cross-linking, mispairing, or strand breaks of the DNA. These drugs are most active in rapidly dividing cells. Common alkylating agents include cyclophosphamide, ifosfamide, carmustine, dacarbazine, and temozolomide. These drugs are mutagenic, teratogenic and carcinogenic. Additionally they can lead to sterility. Other adverse effects include suppression of bone marrow, decreased leukocytes, ulcers, alopecia, nausea, etc. Cyclophosphamide can interact with allopurinol, barbiturates, phenytoin, and warfarin. Ifosfamide can cause myelosuppression and have an increased toxicity when used with other nephrotoxic drugs.

Mechanism of Action of Taxane Drug Class

Paclitaxel and **docetaxel** are examples of taxanes. Paclitaxel and docetaxel are used largely as anti-neoplasia agents. Their mechanism of action is very similar; they both act through inhibition of microtubule activity. Microtubules function by constantly growing and shrinking, and by hyper-activating or inhibiting either the growing or shrinking step of microtubules, mitosis can be inhibited. Paclitaxel and docetaxel inhibit microtubule disassociation during mitosis. Microtubules are important in lining up sister chromatids across the central plane of the cell during metaphase, as well as separating the sister chromatids toward opposite polar ends during anaphase. Paclitaxel and docetaxel block this process, thus retarding tumor growth, and inducing apoptosis. Since paclitaxel and docetaxel inhibit mitosis, these drugs can affect any replicating class of cells including reproductive cells. Other adverse reactions of paclitaxel include nausea, anemia, infection susceptibility due to bone marrow damage, pain in joints, numbness in limbs, and loss of hair. Docetaxel, along with side effects observed with paclitaxel, can cause increased edema.

Anti-Viral Agents Used to Treat Herpes Simplex Virus, Varicella Zoster Virus, and Cytomegalovirus

Acyclovir, valacyclovir, famciclovir are three anti-viral agents that are approved by the FDA to treat infections of the herpes simplex virus and varicella zoster virus. Acyclovir is activated in response to three phosphorylations, the first of which is performed by the viral thymidine kinase, which allows acyclovir to be viral specific. Acyclovir inhibits viral DNA synthesis by inhibiting DNA polymerase and by inhibiting viral DNA incorporation into the DNA of the host organism. Valacyclovir is biotransformed to acyclovir when taken. Famciclovir is biotransformed to penciclovir with similar effects as acyclovir. Ganciclovir, valganciclovir, cidofovir, and foscarnet are used as treatment against cytomegalovirus. Ganciclovir, valganciclovir, and cidofovir inhibit DNA polymerase of the virus, after activation of the anti-viral agent due to phosphorylation, similar to acyclovir. Foscarnet inhibits DNA polymerase of cytomegalovirus without phosphorylation. Fomivirsen uses antisense technology to down regulate viral mRNA and inhibit viral protein synthesis.

NRTIs

Nucleoside reverse transcriptase inhibitors (NRTIs) are some of the oldest drugs used to treat the HIV virus. NRTIs inhibit HIV viral replication by hindering RNA-dependent DNA polymerase. Drugs in the class include: zidovudine (AZT), lamivudine (3TC), abacavir (ABC), tenofovir (TDF), tenofovir alafenamide (TAF), and emtricitabine (FTC). NRTIs can cause lactic acidosis and hepatomegaly. All NRTIs, except, abacavir, need to renally dose adjusted. Tenofovir requires creatinine-clearance-based renal dose adjustment. Compared to other HIV medication classes, NRTIs have few drug interactions. 3TC and FTC should not be used together. Do not use AZT and d4T together as they can antagonize each other. Typically, a patient has a HIV drug regimen that consists of two NRTIs and one other medication from the integrase strand transfer inhibitor (INSTI) class (most commonly dolutegravir or bictegravir).

NNRTIs

Non-nucleoside reverse transcriptase inhibitors (NNRTIs) stop HIV from replicating by binding to reverse transcriptase. Unfortunately, the HIV virus can easily mutate in such a way that confers resistance to this entire class of drugs. Drugs in this class include: nevirapine (NVP), doravirine, and rilpivirine. NNRTIs require care and close monitoring when administered in the context of hepatic impairment, some needing dose adjustments or alternatives considered. Most drugs in this class are CYP 3A4 inducers or inhibitors and as such can interact with many drugs. Drugs in the class are hepatotoxic. As a pharmacist, it is important to check and monitor for potential drug interactions when a patient is taking NNRTIs.

Protease Inhibitors

Protease inhibitors prevent the HIV virus from being able to cleave polyproteins and instead of forming mature HIV particles, immature particles are formed. The immature particles are considered non-infectious. Drugs in this class include: atazanavir (ATV), lopinavir (LPV), and darunavir (TMC-114). Protease inhibitors have many side effects that can be very distressing to a patient. Common side effects include: hyperglycemia, hyperlipidemia, hypertriglyceridemia, osteonecrosis (especially of the hip joints) and lipodystrophy. Common laboratory values should be monitored regularly after the start of PI therapy. Most drugs in this class are CYP 3A4 inhibitors and as such can interact with many drugs. Adverse effects associated with protease inhibitors include nausea, vomiting, diarrhea, and prolonged QT/PR interval for some drugs.

Mechanism of Action of Biologics

Biologics (i.e., biologic response modifiers) are drugs that may be extracted from natural sources (humans, animals, microorganisms) or may be produced through biotechnology. Biologics may be comprised of sugars, proteins, cells, tissues, and/or nucleic acids. Biologics are often heat sensitive and may become contaminated by pathogenic microbes. Biologics include vaccines, blood products, cells, tissues, recombinant proteins, allergens, and genes. Biologics target genes or proteins, typically cell surface receptors and extracellular proteins. For example, for diseases that involve inflammation, such as rheumatoid arthritis, the biologics target proteins of the immune system to reduce the immune response and inflammation, with different biologics targeting different proteins, such as tumor-necrosis factor (TNF) and interleukin 17 (IL-17). However, targeting the immune system reduces the immune response and increases susceptibility to infection. Most biologics can result in some production of antibodies, but most of these antibodies do not cause negative effects.

Inotropic and Chronotropic Drugs

Inotropic compounds are therapeutic drugs which affect the force of heart muscle contraction, positively (increasing force) or negatively (decreasing force). Milrinone and digoxin are examples of positive ionotropes. While negative ionotropes include β-blockers and calcium channels blockers. **Chronotropic compounds** are therapeutic drugs that affect the heart rate, positively (increasing) or negatively (decreasing) the rate. Examples of a positive chronotope include atropine, while β-blockers are an example of a negative chronotrope.

Sympatholytic Drugs

Sympatholytic drugs are used to treat hypertension by decreasing activity from vasopressor control centers of the sympathetic nervous system. They treat mild to severe hypertension, often secondary to first-line therapy. Drugs in this class include methyldopa and clonidine. Methyldopa (generally reserved for pregnancy-related hypertension) is converted to α-methylnorepinephrine and α-methyldopa, which act on the α-adrenoreceptors of the sympathetic nervous system to reduce the resistance of the vascular system, which lowers blood pressure. Methyldopa, by using an amino acid transporter, can cross the blood-brain barrier and enter to act on the sympathetic nervous system. Adverse effects include lethargy, confusion, hypotension and dizziness. Clonidine acts as a partial agonist to alpha-receptors. After initial rise in blood pressure, clonidine facilitates decreased blood pressure by decreasing heart rate and increasing relaxation of the vascular system. Clonidine crosses the blood-brain barrier directly and is broken down rapidly. When administered orally, two doses a day must be given to maintain therapeutic effects. When administered transdermally, it should be applied once every 7 days. Adverse effects include depression and interactions with antidepressants. Withdrawal symptoms can include increased severe hypertension, rapid heartbeat and headaches.

Beta-Adrenoreceptor Blocking Agents

There is a large number of β-adrenoreceptors on the smooth muscles of the vascular systems, and inhibitors (blockers) of these receptors are important clinically for various cardiovascular conditions. **β-blockers** are most often provided as treatment for heart failure/heart disease. They can act through numerous effects, including lowering heart rate, lowering resistance in the peripheral vascular system and may have effects in the central nervous system as wells. β-blockers can also be us used to decrease incidences of angina as well. Propranolol is one Drug in this class. Propranolol has a 3- to 6-hour half-life and generally decreases hypertension by lessening cardiac output, decreasing the heart rate. β-blockers can affect β-receptors on various tissues, which can lead to adverse effects in the renal system as well as the respiratory system. They can also exacerbate already present bradycardia as well as asthma. Withdrawal symptoms include rebound hypertension and rapid heart rate. The drug should be tapered down. Other drugs in this class include metoprolol, nadolol, betaxolol, atenolol, bisoprolol, pindolol, labetalol, acebutolol, penbutolol esmolol (IV only), and carvedilol.

DIGOXIN

Digoxin is a pressor/inotrope and is often used to treat atrial fibrillation (as an adjunct) and paroxysmal atrial tachycardia. Digoxin acts by binding to and inhibiting the Na+/K+ pump on myocytes of the heart, which leads to an increase of intracellular Na+, and this in turn can lead to an increase of intracellular calcium through an increase of Na+/Ca+ exchange. This increase in calcium leads to an increase in contractions of the heart muscle. Digoxin also increases activity of the vagal nerve, which increases AV node activity. Dosing is weight-specific and must consider renal function and other drugs being taken. Adverse effects that signal digoxin toxicity include severe headache, severe tiredness, irregular heart rates, abnormally slow or fast heart rate, hallucinations, and vision problems. More common adverse effects include decreased appetite, mild fatigue, dizziness, decreased libido, and enlarged breasts in males.

MECHANISM OF ACTION OF LOOP DIURETICS

Diuretic drugs are used to control fluid and electrolyte balances in the body which are important in the treatment of many disorders including congestive heart failure and hypertension. By inhibiting NaCl reabsorption at the thick ascending limb of the loop of Henle, loop diuretics can inhibit water reabsorption, leading to the excretion of greater amounts of water via urination. Common loop diuretics include furosemide, torsemide, and bumetanide. These drugs are rapidly absorbed with the effect lasting from 2–6 hours depending on the drug. Adverse effects can include hypokalemia, hypouricemia, hypomagnesemia, as well as severe dehydration and hyponatremia.

Review Video: Diuretics
Visit mometrix.com/academy and enter code: 373276

MECHANISM OF ACTION OF ASTHMA DRUGS

The mechanisms of action of common asthma drugs are described below:

- **Corticosteroids**: Decrease inflammation in the bronchioles of the lungs. Adverse effects include cough and oral thrush. At high doses it can cause thinning of the skin, suppression of growth, suppression of the adrenal gland.
- **Short-acting β2 agonists (LABAs)**: Within minutes, causes relaxation of smooth muscles, inhibiting constriction of the bronchiole tubes and resulting in bronchodilation. Effects last 4–6 hours. These are used for acute asthma exacerbations
- **Long-acting β2 agonists (LABAs)**: Onset is slightly slower than SABA, but similarly causes relaxation of the smooth muscles, inhibiting constriction of the bronchiole tubes and may also inhibit release of histamine by mast cells. Effects last for 12–24 hours so this is a maintenance therapy. Adverse effects include rapid heartbeat, skeletal muscle spasms/shaking; can also lose effectiveness after a week if taken every day. LABAs should not be used without a concomitant inhaled corticosteroid (ICS) therapy because they do not impact underlying airway inflammation in the way ICSs do.
- **Leukotriene modifiers**: These drugs inhibit 5-lipoxygenase, LTD4 and LTE4, which inhibit the activity of leukotrienes, which have been implicated in inflammation of asthma. Adverse reactions include increased bleeding, nausea, allergic reactions, and liver problems. These are not first-line therapy, as inhaled corticosteroid therapy is preferred.

Anticoagulants

Indirect thrombin inhibitors interact and enhance the activity of the protein antithrombin, which can lead to anticoagulant effects. A common drug of this class is known as heparin. Heparin is used to reduce blood clotting. The greatest adverse effect in response to Heparin is excessive bleeding. Heparin is contraindicated in people with bleeding disorders such as hemophilia or thrombocytopenia. **Direct thrombin inhibitors** work by binding directly to the thrombin receptors. These drugs include dabigatran, bivalirudin, and argatroban. They are used to treat thrombosis and heparin-induced thrombocytopenia. Adverse effects are similar to indirect thrombin inhibitors. **Other anticoagulant drugs** include warfarin, which induces its anti-coagulant effects by inhibiting vitamin K and inhibiting prothrombin and clotting factors VII, IX, and X. Warfarin can cause hemorrhaging in an unborn fetus; warfarin can lead to bleeding disorders and skin necrosis and interacts with numerous drugs and herbal products.

Benzodiazepines and Barbiturates

Benzodiazepines and barbiturates bind to the gamma-aminobutyric acid (GABA) receptors on the surface of neuronal cells in the central nervous system (CNS). GABA hyperpolarizes neuronal cells, inhibiting the propagation of action potentials in the CNS. By binding the GABA receptor, benzodiazepines act synergistically with GABA, increasing the efficiency and effect of the neurotransmitter. Barbiturates increase the time that GABA receptors remain open. At higher doses barbiturates mimic GABA effects directly. Benzodiazepines and barbiturates have important sedative effects and can induce sleep. These drugs are used as anesthesia at higher doses. The drugs can also act as anti-seizure medicines. They can depress respiratory and cardiac functions, which at higher doses or when used with opioids can become problematic. These drugs are addictive and it is easy for a patient to become dependent on them. Additionally, the body becomes tolerant to the effects of these drugs, which could cause a rebound effect, leading to insomnia if higher doses are not used. Benzodiazepines include diazepam, lorazepam, triazolam, clobazam, clonazepam, midazolam, and alprazolam. Barbiturates include pentobarbital, secobarbital, and phenobarbital.

Mechanism of Action of Antiepileptic Drugs

Carbamazepine, which can be provided as normal or extended-release forms. Carbamazepine acts by inhibiting voltage channels on nerve cells, inhibiting depolymerization and action potential formation. Does not impair cognitive function. Can cause dizziness, headache, impaired vision, decreased motor skills, and drowsiness. Is used to treat partial seizures and general seizures but does not treat absence seizures. **Oxcarbazepine** and **lamotrigine** are thought to inhibit seizures by blocking sodium voltage channels, inhibiting the production of action potentials. Lamotrigine specifically inhibits action potential in neurons that synthesize the excitatory neurotransmitters of glutamate and aspartate. Oxcarbazepine and lamotrigine can be used to treat partial seizures. Lamotrigine also can be used to treat tonic-clonic seizures. Ethosuximide which is used to treat absence seizures. **Ethosuximide** mechanism of action is not entirely understood, but inhibits the formation of the neurotransmitter, GABA. Side effects include nausea, emesis, dizziness and headaches. Side effects include insomnia, drowsiness, dizziness, headache, and ataxia. Can also lead to severe skin problems and rashes.

Importance of Storage Directions for Insulin

Insulin is an important polypeptide that regulates glucose levels in the blood. In type I diabetes mellitus, insulin levels are lower than normal or absent, and thus replacement insulin must be injected subcutaneously in order for the patient to be able to survive. Glucose is the central component of ATP synthesis and is very necessary for cellular function. Historically porcine insulin was used to treat type I diabetes. Insulin is now made synthetically, by transfecting the human insulin gene into bacteria. There are also many types or analogs of insulin that have been developed including a fast-acting analog known as Lispro. Some unopened insulin should be kept in the refrigerator before use, so attention to storage instructions is important. Depending on the type of insulin being used, there are a specific number of days after opening the insulin that it can be kept at room temperature. Check insulin for unusual cloudiness or particulates. Some insulin is cloudy and some is clear, therefore it is important to counsel a patient about what their specific insulin should normally look like. Do not use insulin past the expiration date.

Pancrelipase

Pancrelipase is a prescription drug that combines three digestive enzymes: lipase, protease, and amylase. Normally produced in the pancreas, these enzymes are important for digestion. During periods of decreased pancreas functionality, this drug can be administered as replacement for the normal enzymes to facilitate digestion. Pancrelipase is often administered in patients with exocrine pancreatic insufficiency. This drug is administered by mouth and the delayed-release tablets should not be crushed or broken. Side effects of this drug can include diarrhea, abdominal pain, nausea, and pain surrounding the anus. Other side effects can include mild anemia, hyperuricemia, and mouth ulcers.

SSRIs

Selective serotonin-reuptake inhibitors (SSRIs) are a type of drug that are used to treat depression, anxiety and other chemical imbalances that might lead to other mental illnesses such as personality disorders. This class of antidepressants inhibits enzymes that lead to the reuptake of serotonin into the presynaptic cleft of the neuron, which leads to an increase of extracellular serotonin levels and increased binding of serotonin to its receptor. This leads to selective activation of serotonin neurons, which is why it is thought that SSRIs tend to show fewer side effects than other antidepressants. It is thought that lower levels of neuron activity can lead to increased depression and anxiety, although exact causes of these mental disorders are not entirely understood. Side effects of SSRIs include nausea, drowsiness, changes in weight, changes in libido, possible panic attacks and liver and kidney problems. SSRIs can also lead to various cardiac events such as arrhythmias, tachycardia, etc. These drugs include citalopram, escitalopram, paroxetine, and fluoxetine.

Tricyclic Antidepressants

Tricyclic antidepressants **(TCAs)** were the first generation of antidepressants. First used in the 1950s, TCAs' mechanism of action is not entirely understood, but it is thought that it might inhibit the reuptake of numerous neurotransmitters including norepinephrine, dopamine and serotonin by neurons. Due to its non-selectivity, these antidepressants, have numerous side effects and are used less now than other antidepressants. Adverse reactions include severe cardiac problems, and overdose of the drug is often fatal. Other side effects include difficult urination, constipation, dry mouth and blurred vision. TCAs are used sparingly to treat depression, neuronal-based pain and chronic bed-wetting. The TCA class includes imipramine, desipramine, trimipramine, clomipramine, amitriptyline, nortriptyline, protriptyline, and doxepin.

MAOIs

Monoamine oxidase inhibitors (MAOIs) are used to treat depression or anxiety in unique cases when these conditions are resistant to other forms of therapy. MAOIs inhibit the activity of the enzyme monoamine oxidase. Monoamine oxidase breaks down neurotransmitters including melatonin, serotonin, epinephrine, dopamine and norepinephrine. MAOIs have numerous side effects, including, when taken by mouth, they can lead to the down-regulation of important metabolic pathways and can lead to a dangerous hypersensitivity event. MAOIs interact with numerous drugs and have important side effects including: anxiety, euphoria, urine retention, rashes, and hypernatremia. MAOIs include isocarboxazid, phenelzine, tranylcypromine, and selegiline. Many food products and natural products have MAOI activity, which can interact with many drugs and should be taken with caution. It is important to counsel patients about which foods can potentially interact with MAOIs.

Haloperidol

Haloperidol **(Haldol)** was one of the first of the major antipsychotics to be developed and is used to control mental/emotional disorders such as schizophrenia, Tourette's syndrome, and involuntary muscle spasms and tics. Haloperidol belongs to the group of the butyrophenone compounds which are known to block dopamine receptors. There are many other forms of drugs in this class of drugs including droperidol, melperone, and lenperone. Haloperidol is probably the most widely used. Haloperidol deaconate is a long-acting form of haloperidol which can be injected once every four weeks at a dose of 50–200 mg, with the first injection no more than 100 mg. Oral drugs can also be administered at a dose of 100 mg per day. Adverse effects include development of tardive dyskinesia, which is a neurological disorder that may occur in response to the long use of dopamine receptor antagonists which can lead to an increase in involuntary movement such as Parkinson-like symptoms. Other side effects include neuroleptic malignant syndrome which can be fatal. Other side effects can include weight gain, drowsiness, muscle-cramps, and severe depression.

Drug Binding

Drug binding occurs when drug molecules enter the blood stream for distribution and bind to protein molecules in the blood in reversible bonds. The most prevalent protein molecule is albumin, but all protein molecules are considerably larger in size than drug molecules and are too large to go through capillary pores and are, therefore, retained in the bloodstream, so drug molecules that are bound to protein are not available to the tissues, limiting the distribution of the drug. The strength of the attraction between a drug molecule and a protein may vary, and this can affect the percentage of drug molecules that are bound to proteins. For example, the attraction between proteins and warfarin is very strong (99% is bound), but some drugs, such as gentamicin (10% is bound) have a very weak attraction and only a small percentage is bound. Thus, only part of drug molecules is bound at any one time. Additionally, drug molecules may compete for binding sites, with one drug molecule replacing another, sometimes resulting in an increase in concentration of one drug to toxic levels.

Adverse Effects, Side Effects, and Interactions

Adverse Effects of Drug Classes

Drug Class	Adverse Effects
Beta-adrenergic antagonists (blockers)	Adverse effects include bradycardia, AV heart block, rebound cardiac excitation, heart failure, postural hypotension, cough-variant asthma, and bronchoconstriction.
HMG-CoA reductase inhibitors (Statins)	Adverse effects include myopathy, rhabdomyolysis, hepatotoxicity, hyperglycemia, memory loss and confusion.
Antidepressants (SSRIs)	Adverse effects include sexual dysfunction, weight gain, serotonin syndrome (altered mental status, myoclonus, incoordination, hyperreflexia, diaphoresis, fever, tremor), and withdrawal syndrome (nausea, dizziness, anxiety, tremor, dysphoria) with abrupt discontinuation.
Antidepressants (TCAs)	Adverse effects include orthostatic hypotension, anticholinergic effects (dry mouth, constipation, blurred vision, dysuria, tachycardia), diaphoresis, sedation, seizures, hypomania, suicidal ideation, and cardiac toxicity with dysrhythmias.
Angiotensin-converting enzyme inhibitors (ACEIs)	Adverse effects include hypotension with first dose caused by vasodilation, cough, hyperkalemia, renal failure, life-threatening angioedema, and fetal injury.
Glucocorticoids/Corticosteroids (Steroids)	Adverse effects involve multiple body systems: Cardiovascular (heart failure, edema, hypertension, electrolyte imbalances), neurological (headache, vertigo, mood swings, depression, seizures, insomnia), endocrine (Cushing's syndrome, growth suppression, dysmenorrhea, hyperglycemia, carbohydrate intolerance), gastrointestinal (pancreatitis, peptic ulcers, esophagitis, abdominal distention), skin (fragility, petechiae, ecchymosis, hirsutism, urticaria, erythema, and impaired healing), musculoskeletal (weakness, loss of muscle mass, osteoporosis), eyes (glaucoma, cataracts), and weight gain.
Opioids	Adverse effects may involve multiple body systems: Cardiovascular (hypotension, flushing, bradycardia), neurological (sedation, disorientation, dizziness, euphoria, dysphoria, confusion, delirium), gastrointestinal (nausea, vomiting, constipation, biliary tract spasm), urinary (retention), skin (rash, pruritus), and respiratory (depression and exacerbation of asthma). Patients may also develop tolerance and become addicted to opioid drugs.

FDA Pregnancy Risk Factor Categories of Prescription and Non-Prescription Drugs

The FDA Pregnancy Risk Factor Categories (ABCD and X) of prescription and non-prescription drugs are as follows:

- **Category A:** Properly controlled studies in pregnant women do not demonstrate developmental abnormalities of the unborn fetus.
- **Category B:** Risk to the fetus was not observed in animal studies, but wasn't performed in controlled studies on pregnant women, or animal studies indicate an adverse effect on fetal development, however, this was not supported by controlled human female studies.
- **Category C**: Animal studies indicate adverse effects on fetus and there are no controlled studies in women or studies on fetal development were not performed in animals or pregnant women.
- **Category D:** Evidence suggests a significant level of risk to the development of a human fetus, but may be acceptable, if the benefit outweighs the risks. I.e. Drugs will save the life of the mother.
- **Category X:** Animal and/or human studies indicate high levels of fetal abnormalities. No benefit ever outweighs the risk. Drugs in this category are contraindicated in pregnant women and in women who may become pregnant.

Teratogenic Effects of Acitretin, Cocaine, Ethanol, Misoprostol, and Vitamin A

The teratogenic effects of these drugs are explained below:

- **Acitretin**: A drug used for psoriasis, an immune-mediated dermatologic disease that leads to formation of lesions on the skin. Exposure to the fetus during the first trimester can lead to general malformations of the limbs and bone structures.
- **Cocaine**: Generally, an abused recreational drug, it can lead to miscarriage, premature birth, as well as abnormal development of various organ systems in the fetus including the heart, digestive system, renal system and the nervous system.
- **Ethanol**: Generally, an abused recreational drug that can lead to Fetal Alcohol Syndrome of the fetus, which is indicative of various abnormalities including malformations of bone structure and organ systems. Children with this disorder often have stunted growth, learning disabilities, and poor motor skills.
- **Misoprostol**: Following exposure to this drug, fetuses have developed facial and skull malformations. Also, this drug increases likelihood of aborted fetus or miscarriages during pregnancy.
- **Vitamin A**: Can lead to multiple side effects including developmental problems of the central nervous system, eyes, ears, cardiac system, and skeletal system.

Cholinergic Crisis

The cholinergic crisis occurs in response to over-stimulation of the neuro-muscular junctions, excess acetylcholine leads to increased activation of the muscarinic receptors. This excess of acetylcholine is generally due to an inhibition of the acetylcholine esterase enzyme. The acetylcholine esterase enzyme is important in the breakdown of acetylcholine. With excessive acetylcholine, the muscarinic receptors become saturated and the muscles do not function with increasing levels of acetylcholine. This can lead to a reduction in muscle tone, increased paralysis, and respiratory depression. Cholinergic crisis can be caused by certain drugs as well as organophosphate poisonings. The antidote of a cholinergic crisis is atropine. Atropine is a competitive inhibitor of acetylcholine and can reverse the cholinergic crisis.

Drugs That Can Influence Insulin Activity

It is important to counsel diabetic patients that certain **drugs can interact with insulin**. This decreases the effect of insulin and leads to increased blood-glucose levels, causing hyperglycemia. Such drugs that decrease the effects of insulin include: anti-HIV drugs, albuterol, asparaginase, calcitonin, corticosteroids, cyclophosphamide, danazol, dextrothyroxine, diazoxide, diltiazem, diuretics, dobutamine, epinephrine, estrogens, ethacrynic acid, isoniazid, lithium, morphine, niacin, nicotine, oral birth control pills, phenytoin, somatropin, and thiazide diuretics. Additionally, certain drugs can also increase insulin activity, leading to decreased glucose levels in the blood causing hypoglycemia. Such drugs that increase the activity of insulin include: ACE inhibitors, alcohol, steroids, beta-blockers, calcium supplements, clonidine, disopyramide, fluoxetine, lithium, guanethidine, MAO inhibitors, mebendazole, pentamidine, phenylbutazone, salicylates, somatostatin, and tetracyclines.

Drug-Drug Interactions

Fluoxetine and phenelzine	Both drugs increase serotonin levels, which can result in life-threatening serotonin syndrome with hyperthermia, tremors, diarrhea, agitation, hypertension, tachycardia, seizures, and rhabdomyolysis.
Digoxin and quinidine	Quinidine doubles the digoxin concentration, placing the patient at risk of life-threatening digoxin toxicity with confusion, dysrhythmia, tachycardia, nausea, omitting, diarrhea, anorexia, and vision changes.
Potassium chloride and spironolactone	Spironolactone (a potassium-sparing diuretic) and potassium chloride can result in life-threatening hyperkalemia with ventricular arrhythmias leading to cardiac arrest, weakness with ascending paralysis and hyperreflexia, diarrhea, and confusion.
Clonidine and propranolol	Because both drugs have similar antihypertensive effects, the additive result can be marked hypotension and bradycardia with the patient experiencing dizziness and risk of fainting.
Theophylline and ciprofloxacin	Ciprofloxacin reduces the clearance of theophylline, resulting in theophylline toxicity with anorexia, nausea, irritability, anxiety, headaches, seizure, and tachycardia.
Methotrexate and probenecid	Probenecid competes with methotrexate for elimination through the kidneys so the methotrexate level increases with pallor, bruising, bleeding, weakness, nausea, vomiting, blood in the stool, decreased urination or anuria, and mouth sores.

Idiosyncratic Reactions

Idiosyncratic reactions refer to abnormal reactions in an organism in response to various compounds such as drugs. The underlying causes of an idiosyncratic reaction are poorly understood, but it is thought that they are largely due to some form of a hypersensitivity that is independent of immune reactions. This indicates that individual might react differently to a drug or toxin due to some genetic polymorphism that is found in a subset of the human population. An example of an idiosyncratic reaction are people who suffer from Phenylketonuria (PKU), a genetic polymorphism by which a there is a deficiency in phenylalanine hydroxylase, which is necessary to metabolize phenylalanine. People with this disorder who ingest phenylalanine can have seizures and other reactions, not normally associated with the ingestion of this amino acid.

Drug Discovery and Development

Development of Theoretical Drugs

The five major steps in the development of a theoretical drug are described below:

1. The first step in drug development is the **identification of a therapeutic target** (i.e. identification of a gene or protein that may have a therapeutic benefit).
2. The second step is to **test the target** through variable experiments such as knockout transgenic mice, in-vitro experiments etc. to determine if the gene or protein will act as a valid target.
3. The third step is to **perform high throughput screening** of compounds to determine any that might interact and inhibit or activate the said target (depending on which is desired), identifying the lead compound.
4. The fourth step is **to use medicinal chemistry techniques to adapt the lead compound** in order to increase its permeability, efficacy and safety.
5. If the compound shows promise it can be moved into the final step of drug discovery and the **compound can be studied further in pre-clinical trial** with hopes of moving to clinical trials, if the compound is safe and effective.

Avenues of Drug Discovery

There are several avenues in which new drugs, compounds, and treatments are discovered. One of the original **avenues for drug discovery** was through the screening of natural products, generally through in vitro and in vivo biological assays to test the therapeutic potential. Several compounds such as salicylic acid and ergotamine alkaloids have been discovered through these means. Other avenues include high- throughput random screening of synthetic compounds; this is when a large amount of random synthetic compounds are screened simultaneously. This is a relatively inefficient way to discover lead compounds for drug discovery. Drug design can also be targeted using such techniques as QASR, as well as by studying possible metabolites of clinically available drugs in order to develop new possible compounds. Another avenue of drug discovery is from observing side effects of other drugs. If a drug provided an unknown yet beneficial side effect, these drugs could be developed further for a new therapeutic use. An example of this is can be observed with the discovery of Viagra.

Rational Drug Design

Historically drugs have been discovered either by accident or by trial and error. While most of the drugs in use today were discovered that way, it has proven not to be an efficient means of drug development, as well; the safety and efficacy profile of drugs found by this way are not usually optimal. **Rational drug design** is a relatively new technique which uses various computational modeling techniques to extrapolate the optimal binding of a compound to a receptor. Rational design generally begins with an understanding of a disease state, a specific receptor for example, in which the drug is designed. Rational drug design is a means to decrease side effects and increase safety and efficacy, while increasing therapeutic specificity of the drug.

Toxic Effects

Immediate vs. Delayed Toxicity

Immediate toxicity can be described as a toxic response that occurs immediately after a single administration of a toxic agent. A high dose of cyanide will lead to a relatively immediate death of an organism after ingestion for example. **Delayed toxicity** can be described as a toxic response that does not occur until a much longer elapsed period of time has passed since the administration of the toxic agent. Carcinogens are great example of delayed toxicity, in which people generally do not show symptoms of any toxic response for twenty to thirty years after administration.

Categories of Bioterrorism Diseases/Agents

Categories of bioterrorism diseases/agents set by the Center for Disease Control are as follows:

- **Category A**: Bioterrorism agents with the highest priority to treat. Healthcare officials must be ready to address any possible outbreak that may occur in the United States. Category A agents are generally considered easily transmitted and can lead to high levels of mortality, which could lead to widespread panic. Such agents include anthrax, plague, botulism, and smallpox.
- **Category B**: Bioterrorism agents with the second highest priority to treat that are only moderately contagious and lead to only moderate levels of illness and lower levels of death. Category agents include ricin, salmonella outbreaks, Q fever, and typhus fever.
- **Category C**: Deals with the possible emergence of infectious diseases that might be engineered and used as a bioterrorism agent. Generally due to the ease of production and transmission into the population, agents of this category might lead to high levels of illness and death.

Chemical Agents Used as Bioterrorism

The following are chemical agents that can be used as bioterrorism:

- **Nerve agents**: Block the acetylcholinesterase enzyme, leading to increased activation at muscarinic and nicotinic receptors. They can cause massive paralysis, seizures, irregular heart beat and severe respiratory distress/failure. Treatment includes atropine to rescue effects of overactive muscarinic receptors and pralidoxime to reverse inhibition of acetylcholinesterases. Diazepam or lorazepam can also be administered for treatment of seizures. Agents include sarin, soma, and VX.
- **Blister agents**: Seriously irritating to the epidermis, as well as mucosal linings and the eyes. These compounds are absorbed quickly through eyes and skin. They can also be inhaled leading to respiratory distress and can lead to severe painful blisters. Agents include sulfur and nitrogen mustards.
- **Blood agents**: Include arsine, an arsenic agent, and cyanide agent, which generally are carried through the blood to various organ sites, leading to organ failure, such as kidney failure. Agents include arsine and hydrogen cyanide.
- **Choking agents**: Include ammonia, chlorine, and phosgene, which can cause irritation of eyes and lungs, uncontrollable coughing, edema, and can be severely life damaging. There is no direct antidote, fresh air, flushing of contaminated areas of the body, treatment of symptoms.

Cyanide

A lethal dose of **cyanide** can range as low as 200 mg, though toxic levels can be observed at much lower doses. Cyanide inhibits oxidative phosphorylation, causing the main source of ATP production to halt, leading to glycolysis to start functioning anaerobically, which will quickly cause most cells to stop functioning, since glycolysis alone does not provide sufficient levels of ATP. Early symptoms of cyanide poisoning include dizziness, headaches, increased heart rate, hypertension, and respiratory distress. Later symptoms include convulsions/seizures and coma, and it can also lead to Parkinson-like symptoms and death. Treatment includes administration of oxygen, along with amyl nitrite, sodium nitrite, and sodium thiosulfate. Treatment should be performed immediately after exposure or as soon as possible.

Acute and Chronic Arsenic Toxicity

Arsenic is a rather poisonous metalloid that is often used in pesticides and found naturally as well. Not uncommon for well water to be contaminated with levels of arsenic. Arsenic can inhibit oxidative phosphorylation. Low levels of arsenic can lead to nausea. Higher levels of acute toxicity can lead to emesis (vomiting) of blood, violent burning during urination, swelling of the brain, convulsions, and death. Chronic toxicity symptoms include cancer development of various organs including liver and kidney, changes in skin color, and gangrene (necrosis of tissue). Symptoms can also include pain and numbness as well as degeneration of muscles, leading to decreased motor skills and possibly paralysis and death. Treatment for arsenic poisoning can include administration of activated charcoal or dimercaprol, an antidote for arsenic poisoning.

Acute Iron Poisoning

Iron levels above 500 μg/dL in the blood are considered toxic. Soon after ingestion of the iron, abdominal pain, vomiting, and diarrhea will ensue. Iron toxicity is often marred with liver damage, leading to increased blood levels of various liver enzymes including BUN, AST and ALT. Also, iron toxicity shows increased creatinine, indicating decreased kidney function and increased INR, suggesting possible bleeding problems. Iron toxicity also leads to decreased blood pressure and tachycardia. If untreated or severe enough iron toxicity can cause increased lethargy, seizures, coma and death. Iron is thought to act locally on the gastrointestinal system leading to pain, but can also be taken up by cells leading to the formation of reactive oxygen species, and also inhibit mitochondrial function. Treatment may include whole bowel irrigation as well as administration of deferoxamine, a potent chelator of iron.

Poison Prevention Packaging Act

The Poison Prevention Packaging Act was passed in 1970, which brought about the usage of "safety caps" on medicine bottles and containers. This act was passed to create medicinal containers that were difficult for young children to open. This could inhibit the chance that young children would be able to open medicine packages successfully or in a timely fashion, so that hopefully the bottles could be taken away from them, before the children could accidentally consume dangerous amounts of the drugs. Many over-the-counter drugs require safety caps, including aspirin and ibuprofen. Prescription drugs are also provided in bottles with safety caps.

First Aid Techniques for Various Sites of Poisoning

Poisonings occur relatively frequently. When poisoning occurs, it is wise to call the 24-hour Poison Control Centers to get helpful information about the poison. Additionally, it is wise to call an ambulance or physician after any poisonings. **Emergency first aid steps** can also be applied in the case of poisonings, but should not substituted for professional help. First aid for poisonings includes:

- If poison is **inhaled**: Remove victim from poison to fresh air. Avoid inhaling poison. Open all doors, windows and use ventilation systems to air out area.
- If poison **contacts skin**: Immediately remove clothing, wash skin with copious amounts of water for about fifteen minutes.
- If poison **contacts eyes**: Remove eye glasses or contacts, wash eyes with copious amounts of water from eye wash or from a glass of water. Wash for fifteen to thirty minutes.
- If poison is **ingested**: Give a small glassful of water to victim and call the poison center and 911 for further instructions.

Activated Charcoal After Ingestion of Poison

Activated charcoal is used to absorb poisons. It can lead to emesis (so prophylactic antiemetics are recommended when administering activated charcoal) and can stain clothes and furniture. It is rapid and non-specific, and it can work with many poisons; however, it can also lead to the removal of beneficial drugs as well. Activated charcoal is generally not effective against metals, alcohols, or caustics. Activated charcoal can be purchased over-the-counter.

Pharmacognosy and Dietary Supplements

Crude Drug, Semi-Purified, and Purified Natural Products

A **crude drug** is any naturally derived compound that may be directly administered to someone as a therapeutic treatment. Crude drugs are generally unrefined and can be plants, minerals, bacterial and animal products. The production (harvesting) and selling of crude drugs was the basis for the pharmaceutical industry. Generally the active ingredient in crude products is not well understood. **Semi-purified products** can include extracts, tinctures of natural products, can show effectiveness, however, generally the active ingredient is still not known, or if known is provided mixed with other components. Large amounts of herbal supplements are provided in this fashion. **Purified natural products** are generally a known active ingredient which is extracted and sold as a supplement. For example the active ingredient of turmeric is known as curcumin, which is extracted and sold commercially.

Drugs vs. Dietary Supplements

To be identified as a **drug**, it must be FDA approved. The active compound must be identified and the activity and safety must be assessed in controlled pre-clinical and clinical trials. Additionally, other components of the drug including purity of the drug and other additives are tightly regulated. Finally, if any claims are made about treatment of specific ailment, it is also considered a drug. A **dietary supplement** is not regulated by the FDA, the active ingredient is generally not known, proof of safety and activity is not required, proof that it is not safe must be required before it is removed from the market. Purity or other additives are not regulated, however, no claims to treat a disease are allowed.

Pharmacologically Active Natural Products

Natural products are those that are produced by living systems in nature, such as plants and microbes, although they can also be synthesized. Some authorities include products of all life forms (including wood, for example) but others include only organic compounds that were actually synthesized by a living organism. The two major classes of natural products include:

- **Primary metabolites**: These are compounds that are essential for life processes, such as growth, development, and reproduction. Examples of primary metabolites include folate, fatty acids, amino acids, vitamins, nucleotides, and numerous enzymes, such as dihydrodipicolinate synthase. Primary metabolites are generally produced on a continuous basis.
- **Secondary metabolites**: These are compounds that are produced by plants or microbes as end products of primary metabolites and originally thought of as waste products. However, although they are not essential for primary processes, they may serve in many roles (some as yet undefined). Examples of secondary metabolites include pigments, toxins, pheromones, and receptor antagonists/agonists.

Secondary Metabolites

Common **secondary metabolites** are derived from plants and include:

- **Alkaloids**: Purine alkaloids are produced from amino acids in plants with most containing nitrogen. Purines include caffeine and theophylline. Purines act by blocking adenosine receptors, causing release of neurotransmitters. Tropane alkaloids are the source of CNS stimulants, such as cocaine. Benzylisoquinoline alkaloids are the source for morphine, codeine and other medications. Catharanthus alkaloids are the source for vinblastine and vincristine; and cinchona alkaloids, for quinine. Glucosinolates produce vegetables and spices, such as wasabi, capers, mustard, and cabbage and may have cancer-preventive factors.
- **Terpenoids**: This is the largest group of natural products found in plants. Terpenoids produce isoprene and essential oils Monoterpenes are the source for menthol; and sesquiterpenes, chamomile and feverfew, which has antimigraine properties. Diterpenes produce taxol, the source of paclitaxel.
- **Phenylpropanoids**: Include flavonoids, anthocyanins, and salicylic acid.
- **Polyketides**: Some are used in laxatives and others have antidepressive actions, such as those found in St. John's wort. Polyketides are the source of many flavonoids that are found in fruits and menthol.

Gingko Biloba

Ginkgo biloba is often used to improve memory, although evidence on its effectiveness is mixed. It has also been suggested to treat intermittent claudication, a decrease in blood flow. Ginkgo biloba is thought to act in part through improving blood flow, as an antioxidant, and by inhibiting clotting factors. There is no regulated dose of ginkgo biloba; however, it is recommended that people take 120–240 mg/day. Ginkgo biloba can lead to headaches and vertigo. Ginkgo biloba interacts with various anticlotting/anti-platelet drugs such as aspirin, warfarin, etc. and can lead to increased bleeding and hemorrhaging.

St. John's Wort

St. John's Wort, also called hypericum perforatum, is used as an alternative treatment for depression as well as anxiety. It is thought to act on the CNS by inhibiting reuptake for serotonin, dopamine, and norepinephrine neurotransmitters. Recommended dose (not regulated) 300 mg, three times a day. Adverse effects include gastrointestinal problems, and insomnia. St. John's Wort has many serious drug interactions, including interacting with antidepressants and digoxin, and it can decrease the effectiveness of oral contraceptives.

Asian Ginseng

Asian ginseng is taken to treat fatigue and to increase concentration. It is thought to have effects on the central nervous system. The suggested dose is 200–400 mg three times a day. Major side effects include increased or decreased blood pressure, insomnia, anxiety, and edema. Ginseng should not be given to individuals with unstable blood pressure. Ginseng interacts with anticoagulant drugs (such as warfarin). It should also not be taken with diabetes drugs due to ginseng's ability to alter glucose levels.

Garlic

Garlic is used for cholesterol and prevention of clogged arteries. Garlic is thought to have anticoagulant, antioxidant, and cholesterol lowering effects. The recommended dose is 600–900 mg/day of freeze-dried supplements. Side effects include bad breath, heartburn, and allergic skin rashes. Garlic can interact with antiplatelet drugs including aspirin and warfarin and should not be taken with the HIV drug Saquinavir.

Echinacea Purpurea

Echinacea is used to treat upper respiratory infections (common cold). Echinacea is thought to possibly help modulate the immune response to help fight mild infection. A dose of 900–1000 mg is recommended, although it depends on the form of echinacea. It is also recommended to take as soon as the cold or other infections begin. Adverse effects can include allergic reactions. This supplement should be used cautiously by people with autoimmune disorders or IgE hypersensitivity reactions (allergic reactions). Echinacea interacts with immunosuppressive agents.

Kava

Kava is used to treat stress in part through increased activation of the GABA receptor. Can interact with Benzodiazepines and barbiturates as well as alcohol. Side effects can lead to decreased motor reflexes similar to alcohol. Machinery should not be operated on kava. Kava can also lead to dry skin and eyes, and liver disease and jaundice if taken excessively. Should not be taken with present liver disease/failure. The dose is 70–250 mg a day divided into 2–3 doses.

Flavonoids

Flavonoids occur naturally in plant products such as soy and have many biological effects particularly anti-oxidant effects. Anti-oxidants have important protective properties of cells, by neutralizing reactive oxygen species. These compounds are thought to reduce risk for heart disease, cancer, and inflammation. Important flavonoids include quercetin, resveratrol and epicatechin, which can be found in onions/apples, tea/cocoa, and red wine respectively. The bioavailabilities of flavonoids are variable, and it is unclear if they possess any valid therapeutic effects. It is thought that a large amount of food products would need to be eaten to reach therapeutically effective doses of the flavonoids. Flavonoids are generally considered healthy, however, if taken at high doses, as some studies have found, flavonoids may act as a pro-oxidant, leading to greater cell damage. Flavonoids, like anything else, if taken, must be taken in moderation and not as a replacement for a healthy diet and exercise.

Herbal Interactions with Warfarin

The following **herbals interact with Warfarin**, causing the below effects:

- **Danshen (Salvia miltiorrhiza)**: Commonly used in Chinese herbal medicine as a remedy for cardiac issues. It is widely been reported to increase blood "thinning" and decrease blood clotting. It can interact and exacerbate the effects of warfarin.
- **Garlic**: Used to as a treatment for atherosclerosis, can exacerbate warfarin effects.

- **Ginkgo biloba**: Evidence suggests it can decrease clotting, can exacerbate warfarin effects.
- **Ginseng**: Can decrease effects of warfarin.
- **St. John's Wort**: Evidence indicated may decrease the bioavailability of warfarin.

Dietary Health Supplement and Education Act

The Dietary Health Supplement and Education Act was passed in 1994, which stated various regulations of dietary supplements. A dietary supplement must be labeled as such, and must contain vitamins, minerals, amino acids, or other botanical agents, besides tobacco, which can be ingested orally. The Food and Drug Administration (FDA) regulates these supplements as food products and not as drugs. While drugs are approved only if safety and an effective use can be proven, dietary supplements are only regulated by the FDA if they have been proven harmful. For it to be considered as a dietary supplement, it also cannot be marketed as a meal itself. As dietary supplements, they cannot make claims that it can treat any disorder. If they make these claims, it is in violation of federal law and would be considered an illegal drug, since the FDA did not approve the supplement to treat such disorders. The Dietary Health Supplement and Education Act allows people to choose what they consume, however, there are no true regulations in place to control these substances, which can still lead to the possibility of harmful drugs and compounds reaching the public.

Pharmaceutics/Biopharmaceutics

Dosage Form and Drug Release

The following are several ways medications are released:

- **Delayed release**: Enteric coated tablets. Generally, enteric coating wears off in the duodenum and once coating is dissolved the drug dissolves completely.
- **Prolonged release**: The form of a drug that takes slightly longer to absorb into the bloodstream. These drugs are sometimes called delayed release drugs.
- **Sustained release**: A drug that releases a small initial amount of drug and then releases the rest of the drug over 12–24 hours. The goal of sustained release drugs is to provide more consistent drug levels in the body.
- **Extended release**: Essentially the same as a sustained release drug.
- **Controlled release**: Essentially the same as a sustained or extended release drugs. Controlled release drugs release the drug continuously with the goal of consistent plasma levels that vary minimally.

Extended or Controlled Release Tablets

There are several types of tablets that release medication over a period of time or delay release of medication. Some **controlled release drugs** are use multiple small pellets instead of one large pellet. Small pellets reduce the chance of dosage failure, help for a more uniform distribution across the GI tract, and may increase risk for dose dumping. These types of **tablets release their drug contents via three mechanisms:** diffusion, erosion and osmosis.

- **Diffusion tablets** release their drugs slowly across a membrane once they come in contact with gastric juices.
- **Erosion tablets** are coated with a special coating that dissolves (or at times are an entire tablet that dissolves) extremely slowly, therefore releasing the drug slowly.

- **Osmosis based tablets** have a very small hole drilled on the outside of the tablet where fluid enters the tablet once swallowed. This allows for the osmotic core to push out through the hole and causes the drug to be released slowly. The osmosis core may not dissolve fully and will be excreted in the feces. These are called ghost tablets.

Routes of Drug Administrations

Routes of drug administrations are as follows:

- **Oral administration** of a drug is generally the most common and most popular due to its ease of use and ease of compliance. Oral drugs are generally absorbed in the digestive (gastro-intestinal) system and are used for overall systemic effects.
- **Rectal administration** of a drug is often given locally or for compounds that are normally broken down or inactivated by the digestive system or liver.
- **Parenteral administration** involves the injection of drug using a hypodermic needle. Generally, drugs are given via this administration for rapid absorption and for drugs that can be inactivated by the digestive system and the liver. Routes of administration include subcutaneous (into the skin), intramuscular (into the muscle) and intravenous (into the vein).
- **Topical administration** is generally local, such as an ointment to treat an allergic reaction. Systemically topical routes of administration do not work well due to poor absorption, although some patches exist which do this, such as the nicotine patch.
- **Respiratory route of administration** is a good site for rapid drug absorption and is good for the treatment of asthma. It is also used for other drugs due to the rapid systemic absorption from the lung.

Inhaled Pulmonary Drug Delivery

Most drugs that are **inhaled either into the lungs or into the nasal passage** are focused on local and not systemic drug delivery. Most often drugs that are inhaled into the lungs are done so to act locally on pulmonary tissue. Examples of medications that act locally in the lungs include albuterol and inhaled steroids. By inhaling steroids (such as fluticasone) into the lungs, a lower dose can be used and there is little systemic absorption. This is especially advantageous when steroid based medications have many side effects when taken orally. While it is generally the goal to not have systemic absorption of inhaled medications, pulmonary tissue can be used to deliver medications systemically. Pulmonary tissue is highly vascularized and has a large surface area. Drugs that are inhaled avoid first pass metabolism, allowing smaller dosages. Recently, inhaled insulin has become available and is inhaled into the lungs and then systemically absorbed.

Inhaled Nasal Drug Delivery

Most drugs that are **inhaled into the nasal passage** are focused on local and not systemic drug delivery. Typical examples of nasal medications include inhaled steroids and inhaled liquid decongestants. The nasal passages have excellent vascularization and as such can be used for systematic drug delivery. Several migraine medications are inhaled through the nasal passage and have a rapid systemic onset. By administering these medications via the nasal passages, first pass elimination is avoided so a lower dose can be used. Additionally, medicines inhaled through this route are rapidly absorbed, so onset time is generally faster. New drug development continues to focus on nasal drug delivery as a viable option for delivery of protein and peptide drugs.

Drugs Absorbed Topically

While the skin is generally viewed as an organ that serves to protect vital organs and mucosal linings, it is susceptible to damage and penetration with the appropriate vehicle. Skin is layered and composed of the epidermis (outermost layer), dermis and subcutaneous fat. **Drugs pass into the skin via passive diffusion.** Drugs that are small and not chemically charged pass into the skin much easier compared to large, polar molecules. The stratum corneum, which is located in the epidermis, is the layer of the skin that limits the speed of drug absorption through the skin. This is because the stratum corneum is the hardest avascular layer of the skin. The viability of a specific area of skin can also affect drug absorption through the skin. Skin tissue that is infected, damaged or burnt has a higher level of drug permeability.

Topical Drug Delivery Forms

Topical drug delivery forms are wide and varied and can include powders, ointments, creams, solutions and various transdermal patches and occlusive dressings. The goal of all of these vehicles is to keep the drug on the skin long enough to allow penetration through the skin. Most patches, occlusive dressings and ointments help prevent water loss and locally increase moisture to the skin. This helps increase the amount of drug that can penetrate into the skin. Solutions are used for areas where a thicker ointment or cream will not work (such as the scalp or groin) and if there is good drug penetration without a thicker vehicle. Powders are used most commonly with wet or weeping skin lesions. The goal of powders is to help evaporate water and dry out a lesion along with delivering local medication. Skin penetration is much less with powders.

Transdermal Patches

Transdermal patches have become a more popular dosage form in the past 10 years. There are now patches for birth control, smoking cessation, pain relief and blood pressure to name a few. In general, patches are composed of an adhesive layer, a drug matrix/reservoir where the drug is housed in a crystalloid material, and a membrane that controls how fast the drug is released into the skin. Medication that is delivered via a transdermal patch does not encounter first pass metabolism and therefore a lower dose can be used to achieve the same clinical effect. Additionally, patches are able to provide a continuous rate of medication delivery, which aids in steady plasma levels.

Counseling Points

Counseling points related to transdermal patches must be tailored the specific patch that is being prescribed. It is important to counsel patients to open and pull the backing off the patch before placing the patch on an area of skin that is free from hair. It is also important to counsel patients to avoid cutting the patch in any form. The patch usually contains a matrix of drug with some type of rate limiting membrane. This membrane must stay intact, if it is cut or torn, it is possible the patch will dose dump, causing potential adverse reactions. It is also important to counsel patients as to the length that the patch should be worn. This is highly variable and depends on the type of patch being used. Patients also need to be counseled to only place one patch on their body at a time.

Fentanyl Patches

It is very important to counsel a patient the first time they are prescribed a **fentanyl patch**. Fentanyl has the potential to cause serious adverse reactions, including respiratory depression and death. A patient should be counseled that only one patch should be applied at a time (unless given a prescription for otherwise) and that it will take about 12–24 hours before onset of pain relief from the drug, with a full duration of 24–72 hours. It is important to make sure that a patient has oral pain medications for pain to utilize until the fentanyl patch reaches a therapeutic level in the bloodstream. Fentanyl patches should be changed every 72 hours. Counsel the patient to fold the old patch in half and flush the patch down the toilet to prevent accidental exposure or misuse. Explain to the patient that they may feel drowsy or dizzy and to not drive until they know how the medication affects them. Remind them to call their doctor or dial 911 immediately if they are having trouble breathing.

Implantable Drug Delivery

Implantable drug delivery is a fast changing and, in many ways, under-utilized drug delivery system. Implantable drug delivery devices are currently being used as long-term birth control in the forms of implantable capsules and as drug releasing IUDs. Implantable drug delivery is also used in cardiac stents. These stents are put in place in the heart and then continue to release a small amount of drug that helps prevent the area from re-clotting. Generally, some type of surgical procedure is required to place an implantable device. Additionally, implantable birth control must be surgically removed after a period of time (usually 3–5 years) and fertility is not immediately restored once the device is removed. In fact, it can take up to a year for fertility to be restored after an implantable device is removed.

Insulin Pumps

Insulin pumps were once cumbersome and rarely used by diabetics. However, in the past few years, insulin pumps have become sleek and small devices that are gaining popularity for their convenience and reliability. Insulin pumps continuously deliver short acting insulin at a level programmed into the device. This essentially mimics basal insulin release in the body. Additionally, they can be programmed to deliver a bolus of insulin to accommodate additional carbohydrate intake during meals. Insulin pumps are attached to a thin tube that contains a small needle. The needle is typically inserted subcutaneously under the skin on the stomach. This covered with a bandage and can stay in place for 3–4 days. Insulin pumps are expensive and can break, making this device not ideal for some patients. Additionally, patients must still monitor their blood sugar carefully to make sure they are not becoming hypo or hyperglycemic.

Rectal and Vaginal Drug Delivery

Typically, **vaginal drug delivery** is used to deliver medicine to local tissue. These agents are usually a cream or ointment that contains antifungal or antiprotozoal medications. Additionally, hormone replacement creams are often applied to internal and external vaginal tissue. These creams provide action to local tissue, but are also absorbed systemically as well. Any medication absorbed via the vagina avoids first pass metabolism. **Rectal drug delivery** is used for systemic and local drug delivery. Typically, rectal formulations or either in a suppository or enema solution form. Rectal drug delivery avoids first pass metabolism if it is absorbed in the lower rectum. If it is absorbed any higher in the intestinal tract, first pass metabolism may or may occur. Drug absorption into rectal tissue is best when the medicine is in a fatty base vehicle such as cocoa butter. The rectum is also used to administer medications such as rectal diastat, which is used to help stop a seizing patient.

Biodegradability and Biocompatibility of Polymers in Drug Preparation

A **polymer** is a macromolecule made from a number of similar monomers (small molecules). Polymers may be natural (proteins, cellulose, DNA) or synthetic (plastics, epoxy). Polymers are used in the formulation of drugs, as they can modulate the drug properties and aid in delivery. Drug polymers must be assessed for both biodegradability and biocompatibility. Drug polymers may be biodegradable, which means that they can decompose, such as in an aerobic or anaerobic environment or through the action of hydrolysis or enzymes during metabolism. The amount of biodegradation and the effect of biodegradation byproducts must be assessed. Other polymers may be nonbiodegradable, such as polyethylene and Teflon. Biocompatibility refers to the ability of a polymer to carry out its intended activity without causing undesirable effects, local or systemic.

Biocompatibility issues include whether a polymer is cytotoxic or may result in allergic response or mutations, and all of these issues must be resolved in testing before a drug comes to market.

Excipients

Almost all tablets manufactured contain some type of **excipient** in addition to the active drug. Fillers are used to make a tablet an appropriate size to manufacture in a large-scale setting. Fillers include: lactose, glucose, cellulose and calcium carbonate. Disintegrants are used to make sure a tablet dissolves when it touches liquid. Disintegrants include: starch, cellulose and sodium starch glycolate. Binders are used to help add strength to the tablet. Binders include: starch, cellulose, gelatin, methyl cellulose. Glidants are added to help particle flow during the manufacturing process. Glidants include: silica, talc and magnesium stearate. Lubricants are added to help tablet formation and improve release from the die wall. Lubricants include: magnesium stearate, polyethylene glycol, stearic acid. Anti-adherents are used to keep the tablet from adhering to the punches. Anti-adherents include: talc, starch and cellulose.

Solid Oral Delivery Dosage Forms

Oral solid dosages are very common due to their convenience. Traditional release of solid dosage forms is a powder, granule, capsule, or tablet taken orally. Powders and granules as a dosage form have an advantage over tablets in that a larger dosage can be given, but a disadvantage is that any unpleasant odor or taste cannot be masked. Extended-release oral dosage forms are capsules. An advantage of extended-release dosage forms is that they maintain relatively constant serum drug concentrations due to their coating. The coating is an enteric, diffusion-controlled reservoir system, diffusion-controlled matrix system, dissolution-controlled system, ion-exchange resin, osmotically controlled system, or complex formation. Capsules are advantageous as oral dosage forms because they can contain multiple active ingredients. The rapid-release products' dosage forms are tablets, strips, or lollipops. Examples of immediate-release tablets are compressed, multicompressed, chewable, buccal, sublingual, and effervescent.

Oral Solution Stability and Common Solution Vehicles

Water is the most common **solvent** used in pharmaceutical solutions. Because drugs are not always completely soluble in water alone, a **cosolvent** is often used. Common cosolvents include ethanol, glycerol, propylene glycol and simple syrup. Additional items added to oral solutions include buffers, density modifiers, isotonicity modifiers, preservatives and agents that increase viscosity, sweeteners and flavors. Each manufactured solution will have an expiration date. It is important to note items that need to be kept refrigerated. If they do not stay cold, it is possible that the stability of the product has been compromised. If a solution has changed color, smell or has become cloudy, it is possible that the solution is no longer stable. Always err on the side of caution: if you are worried that a solution is no longer stable, do not dispense the product to the patient.

Suspensions and Flocculating Agents

Ideally a **suspension** is formulated in such a way that the drug particles in the suspension stay continuously dispersed and do not settle to the bottom of the container. If this cannot be achieved, suspensions must at a minimum be formulated so that the drug particles stay appropriately dispersed in the suspension once it has been shaken. Additionally, **flocculating agents** such as electrolytes, surfactants and polymeric flocculating agents can be used to keep the drug particles from compacting at the bottom of the bottle. Electrolytes change the zeta potential and include phosphates, sodium salts and citrates. Surfactants can change the charge density of the entire system, therefore helping to create a flocculated suspension. Surfactants include polysorbates and sorbitan. Polymeric flocculating agents are used to make a highly flocculated suspension slightly less flocculated. Polymeric flocculating agents include silicates, tragacanth, carbomers and alginates.

Pharmacokinetic Parameters

Rate-Limiting Step for Kinetics of Drug Absorption

The rate-limiting step is the slowest step in the kinetics of a drug's absorption. The rate-limiting step could be the slow release from the formulation (i.e., tablets of poorly water-soluble drugs) or it could be the diffusion through the gastrointestinal wall (highly water-soluble drug that dissolves quickly). Drugs that are poorly water-soluble have very little dissolution of the drug from the tablet's surface. Instead, the tablet must be completely dissolved before being an effective therapy. The Noyes-Whitney equation is the rate of drug dissolution from the solid through the layer that surrounds it into the membrane or circulation.

Drug Shelf-Life Stability

The shelf-life stability varies from dosage form. The shelf-life stability is determined by the Arrhenius equation, where A is the pre-exponential factor or simply the prefactor, R is the gas constant, T is the temperature, and Ea is the activation energy of a chemical reaction with rate constant k.

$$\mathrm{k} = \mathrm{A} \cdot e^{\frac{-E_a}{R \cdot T}}$$

The units of the pre-exponential factor are identical to those of the rate constant and will vary depending on the order of the reaction. If the reaction is first order it has the units s^{-1}, and for that reason it is often called the frequency factor or attempt frequency of the reaction. Most simply, k is the number of collisions which result in a reaction per second.

Dosing on Body Weight

Dosage is calculated on the patient's weight or body surface area. This specific dose is required for pharmaceuticals that have a narrow therapeutic range. In addition, some pharmaceuticals are dosed on the patient's creatinine clearance because it is vital to dose appropriately with the patient's renal ability. When dosing on body weight, either the patient's actual body weight (ABW) or the ideal body weight (IBW) is used. If detailed information is not available, dosages are typically calculated based on a 70 kg individual. If the dosage is to be given to a smaller or larger individual, the typical dose can be multiplied by the ratio of the patient's apparent weight to 70 kg. IBW is calculated as:

IBW in kg = Gender Factor in kg +2.3 kg * (Height in inches-60in)

This gender factor is 50kg for males and 45.5kg for females.

Dosing on body surface area is calculated as:

$$\mathrm{BSA}\ in\ m^2 = \sqrt{\frac{(\mathrm{Height}\ in\ cm) \cdot (\mathrm{Weight}\ in\ kg)}{3600}}$$

The dosing based on creatinine clearance (CrCl) is calculated by the following:

$$\mathrm{CrCl}\ in\ mL/\min = \frac{(140yr - \mathrm{Age}\ in\ yr) \cdot \mathrm{Weight}\ in\ kg}{72\ \cdot \mathrm{Serum\ creatinine}\ in\ mg/dL}$$

Female CrCl is typically 0.85x that of males.

Methods for Dosing Pediatric Patients

There are four main methods of calculating pediatric dose. The first is to calculate the body surface area (based on a chart where the height and weight of the child intersect) divided by the pediatric correction factor (1.73). The second method is Clark's rule for infants and children, where the weight in pounds is divided by a correction factor of 150 and multiplied by the adult dose. The third method is Fried's rule is for children from 1–2 years of age which is calculated by multiplying the age in months by the adult dose divided by a correction factor of 150. The final method for determining dose for pediatric patients is the age of the child in years multiplied by the adult dose and divided by the child's age in years + 12.

Examples of Dosing Calculations

Calculate the dose that would be dispensed to a patient based on a prescription that states the following:

- 50 mg amitriptyline (25 mg tablets are available)
- 37.5 mg dothiepin (75 mg tablets are available)
- 37.5 mg nortriptyline (25 mg tablets are available)
- 0.5 mg digoxin (250 mcg tablets are available)
- 2.5 g neomycin sulfate (500 mg tablets are available)

Answer:

50 mg amitriptyline = 50 mg / 25mg = 2 tablets
37.5 mg dothiepin = 37.5 mg / 75 mg = 0.5 tablet
37.5 mg nortriptyline = 37.5 mg / 25 mg = 1.5 tablets
0.5 mg digoxin = 0.5 mg / 0.25 mg = 2 tablets
2.5 g neomycin sulfate = 2.5 mg / 0.5 mg = 5 tablets

Calculate how many milliliters of codeine phosphate (subcutaneous injection) are required in order for the patient to receive his or her prescribed dose of 35 mg. There is a solution of the drug available at 50 mg per milliliter. Also, the same patient needs a dose of 50 mg of amoxicillin trihydrate (oral). There is a solution available at 125 mg in 5 mL. Calculate the volume needed to provide the patient with the 50 mg dose.

Answer:

The calculation is as follows for **codeine phosphate**:

35 mg codeine phosphate required / 50 mg per mL = 0.7 mL
0.7 mL of the 50 mg/mL solution equals a 35 mg dose

The calculation is as follows for **amoxicillin trihydrate**:

125 mg / 5 mL = 25 mg/mL concentration of available solution
50 mg / 25 mg/L = 2 mL
2 mL of the 125 mg in 5 mL solution equals a 50 mg dose

Calculate the compounded medication to be dosed at 0.4 mg per kg of the patient's actual body weight. The patient weighs 35 kg. The dose is to be given intravenously at a concentration of 0.25 mg/mL.

Answer:

Since the dose is 0.4 mg/kg per day, the dose is calculated below:

$$Daily\ dose = \frac{35\ kg \times 0.4\ mg}{0.25\frac{mg}{mL}} = \frac{14\ mg}{0.25\frac{mg}{mL}} = 56\ mL$$

The patient will receive 56 mL of the drug at a concentration of 0.25 mg/mL daily.

Calculate the compounded medication to be dosed at 1.4 mg per kg of a patient's actual body weight. The patient weighs 80 kg. The dose is to be given intravenously at a concentration of 0.12 mg/mL.

Answer:

Since the dose is 1.4mg/kg, the dose is calculated below:

$$Daily\ dose = \frac{80\ kg \times 1.4\ mg}{0.12\frac{mg}{mL}} = 933.3\ mL$$

The patient will receive 933.3 mL of the drug at a concentration of 0.12 mg/mL.

Drug Delivery

Solubility

Physiochemical properties of drugs related to drug delivery include **solubility**, which refers to the ability of the drug to be dissolved so it can be absorbed into the tissues. The body has two environments of concern, a water (hydrophilic) environment and a lipid (lipophilic) environment. Water is a polar molecule that dissolves polar molecules while lipids are non-polar molecules that dissolve non-polar molecules (like dissolves like). The degree of solubility in water (S_w) is usually reported as a logarithm ($logS_w$), and drugs that are hydrophilic generally have a $logS_w$ ranging from about 0.4 to <0. The degree of solubility in lipids is reported as the logarithm of the partition coefficient (logP). A negative logP indicates poor lipophilic qualities; and positive, high. Hydrophilic and lipophilic properties of a drug must be properly balanced in order for the drug to dissolve and reach the right site of action because cell membranes have both hydrophobic and lipophobic properties. To improve hydrophilicity, polar groups may be added to a compound, it may be changed into a salt, or the method of dispensing the drug changed (such as from oral to IV). Adding non-polar molecules, such as fluorine or chlorine, increases lipophilicity.

Stability

Physiochemical properties of drugs as they relate to drug delivery include **stability**, or the ability of the drug to retain chemical properties, which is a process that is essential to ensure therapeutic action. Stability is based on the rate of changes and the amount of degradation that occur during the chemical reactions of drug metabolism. Drug compounds may degrade through improper storage or administration outside the body and through the action of enzymes inside the body. Chemical reactions that may alter composition include oxidation, which may be caused by exposure of some drugs to light. In order to combat oxidation, drugs may be stored in amber containers or antioxidants included in the drug compound. Hydrolysis may break apart some of the chemical bonds, and this may be positive or negative, depending on the drug. In some cases, hydrolysis may cause a drug to become inactive over time, so frequent dosing or reconstituting powder immediately before administration may be needed to maintain adequate blood levels. Hydrolysis occurs more rapidly with drugs containing esters than those containing amides.

Drug Product Manufacturing

New Chemical Entities

The new chemical entities are preformulation, formulation development, and marketed product. Preformulation is the characterization of the physical and chemical properties of the active ingredient, including the physical attributes, solubility, chemical, and analytical. Formulation development is the ongoing process in the clinical trials for the dosage form of injectable, topical (local and systemic), and oral. The marketed product is the development of the final dosage, which includes the physical attributes (color, shape, size, taste, and viscosity), packaging, production equipment, production site, country of origin (manufacturing), and country of marketing (sold in).

Stages of Drug Development

The main sections of drug development are preclinical drug development, clinical drug development, and postmarketing. The preclinical drug development involves the preclinical PK/PD (mechanism-based models, *in vivo* potency and drug interactions, biomarker and surrogate identification, and dosage form) and the transitional PK/PD (allometric scaling and dose escalation). The clinical drug development encompasses the clinical trials (phases I, II, and III), analytical (characterization of dose-concentration-effect relationship, routes of administration, therapeutic index, food and gender effects, active metabolites, drug interactions, disease interactions, tolerance, and bridging studies). Predictive PK/PD (simulations and trial forecasting) are also part of clinical PK/PD. During postmarketing PK/PD, the postmarketing surveillance is done.

Product Line Extensions and Combination Products

Product line extensions are for NDA-approved drugs in a different dosage strength or dosage form. Regulatory approval is based on analytical and manufacturing controls, stability, bioavailability and bioequivalence studies, and clinical trials. Oral product line extensions (different dosage strength) require bioequivalence studies for registration. However, if a new therapeutic is included in the formulation, it requires new efficacy studies and a new NDA and not a product line extension. Combination products contain at least two regulated components. The components are drug, device, or biologic. Combination products can be at least two separate products packaged together.

Investigational New Drug Document Application

Three sections comprise the Investigational New Drug (IND) application: animal pharmacology and toxicology studies, manufacturing information, and clinical protocols and investigator information. In the first section, preclinical data is collected for determining the relative safety in humans as extrapolated from animals. The manufacturing section of the IND contains the analytical properties of all reagents used to generate the drug, stability of the drug, and controls used to monitor the risk of drug. Risk assessment is an important part of the drug manufacturing process because it monitors and continually improves the consistency of each lot of drug manufactured, thereby maintaining the quality of the drug dispensed. The last section contains the design and implementation for a phase I clinical trial that the sponsor would like to pursue for that drug. This section also provides physicians with the details on the drug and enhances their understanding of the drug's intended use and target patient population.

Pharmacokinetics

Linear Kinetics

Linear kinetics is also known as linear biotransformation or first order kinetics. When a drug follows linear kinetics, how fast the drug is metabolized in the body is directly proportional to the amount of the drug given. If you were to plot this on a graph, you would simply get a linear line that has a slope equal to $-k/2.303$, where k is the first order elimination rate constant. The elimination rate constant and half-life of drugs that follow first order kinetics are independent of the amount of drug given. Most drugs in general follow linear kinetics.

Non-Linear Kinetics

Non-linear kinetics is also known as non-linear biotransformation or zero order kinetics and in general, few drugs exhibit non-linear kinetics as an exclusive form of metabolism. Drugs such as ethanol, phenytoin and salicylates do exhibit exclusive non-linear kinetics. When drugs such as phenytoin follow non-linear kinetics, how fast the drug is metabolized in the body is not directly proportional to the amount of drug given. Non-linear biotransformation of drugs is most commonly due to these drugs needing to be transported via a protein carrier before biotransformation can occur. There are a finite number of protein carriers and therefore these drugs are dependent on how fast they can pass through these protein carriers.

Compartment Models in Pharmacokinetics

Pharmacokinetic models are categorized as either one-compartment open models or multi-compartment models.

- A **one-compartment open model** is used when a drug is given intravenously and makes the assumption that the drug is immediately absorbed and distributed throughout the body. If you were to graph this absorption, it would be a linear line.
- A **two-compartment open model** takes into account that some drugs when administered intravenously, do not absorb into the body in an exactly linear fashion. This model has an initial, brief distribution phase and then a linear elimination phase. This model is only accurate for drugs that are eliminated via a first-order process.
- A **three-compartment open model** works essentially like the two-compartment open model and takes into account that some drugs distribute into deep tissues, which is generally a slow process.

Bioequivalent Drugs

The FDA requires that all generic drugs that would like to come to market have both in vitro and in vivo tests performed to prove that they are equivalent to the bioavailability of the original brand name drug. For a generic drug to be FDA approved as **bioequivalent**, it does not have to be identical in all pharmacokinetic parameters to the original brand drug. It does, however, have to be identical in all parameters that are considered important for proper action of the drug in the body. The FDA gives all generic drugs that enter the market either an A rating or a B rating. Generic drugs with an A rating are considered by the FDA to be bioequivalent to the brand name drug. Generic drugs with a B rating are not considered by the FDA to be bioequivalent by in vivo tests and were instead approved by in vitro tests. These drugs are mostly older drugs and only 3 % of generic drugs are currently B rated.

Bioavailability, Relative Bioavailability, and Absolute Bioavailability

Bioavailability is a measurement that is used to determine the quantity and the speed that an active drug enters circulation and is available to cause a pharmacological effect. Bioavailability is determined for every new drug before the FDA approves that drug. Additionally, bioavailability must be determined for new formulations of previously FDA approved drugs. **Relative bioavailability** is also called apparent bioavailability and is the amount of active drug that is in a specific dosage form that is available for use compared to a known standard. The following equation allows you to determine relative bioavailability:

$$\textbf{Relative bioavailability} = \frac{[\text{AUC}]_A/\text{dose A}}{[\text{AUC}]_B/\text{dose B}}$$

Absolute bioavailability is the amount of drug that is systemically absorbed and pharmacologically active when administered by any route other than IV administration. The following equation allows you to determine absolute bioavailability.

$$\textbf{Absolute bioavailability} = \frac{[\text{AUC}]_{PO}/\text{dose}_{PO}}{[\text{AUC}]_{IV}/\text{dose}_{IV}}$$

Biosimilars

A biosimilar is a medication that is similar to its biologic formulation. The determination of whether a biosimilar is suitable for follow-on protein products is limited. Examples of biosimilars are insulin, growth hormones, and immunologic agents. The issue of biosimilars becomes a household issue when a patient would like to switch to a generic and less expensive form (biosimilar) of the drug they are taking. While the price of a biosimilar is beneficial to patients, these medications may or may not be the best choice for their treatment. The pharmacist should discuss with the patient and the physician any questions about switching to a biosimilar.

Drug Half-Life

The time needed for a drug level to be one half of its original concentration is called the **elimination half-life**. The elimination half-life ($t^{1/2}$) and the elimination rate constant (K) are intimately connected and form the equation $K=0.693/t^{1/2}$. This equation allows you to determine the elimination rate constant of a first order reaction if you know a drug's half-life and conversely determine a drug's half-life if you know the elimination rate constant. A drug's half-life often determines how often a drug needs to be administered. Generally, a drug is considered to be at steady state in the body after approximately 5 half-lives. It is important to remember that drugs often have active metabolites and these metabolites may or may not have similar kinetic properties. The half-life of the original parent drug may or may not be the same as its metabolites.

Volume of Distribution

Volume of distribution **(V_D)** is also known as the apparent volume of distribution. A drug's apparent volume of distribution is a theoretical number that approximates how widely the drug is distributed throughout the body after a drug is given. The V_D of any given drug can be affected by several factors including renal failure, dehydration, shock and blood loss. Additionally, the V_D of many drugs will vary with age. Drugs that are significantly protein bound and generally stay in the vascular compartment have a V_D that is below 10L. Drugs that are not protein bound, lipophilic and move into fatty tissues have a V_D that is well over 15,000L. Drugs with a V_D between these two numbers distribute out of the vascular compartment, but not entirely into fatty tissue. The following equation can be used to determine V_D.

$$V_D = \frac{\textbf{Amount of drug in the body}}{\textbf{Concentration of drug in blood}}$$

Therapeutic Drug Monitoring

Therapeutic drug monitoring is a very important aspect of pharmacokinetics. It is important to remember that all drugs have a therapeutic range as opposed to a finite value. However, some medications such as digoxin, theophylline, lithium, aminoglycosides warfarin and many anti-seizure medications have a very narrow therapeutic range. This means that below its therapeutic range, the drug is ineffective and above, it is potentially toxic. Therapeutic drug monitoring is most importantly focused on drugs that have a narrow therapeutic range. Drugs with a narrow therapeutic range are usually individually dosed and are closely monitored by a patient's physician and pharmacist. Most drugs in this class have laboratory tests that can be performed to get patient specific drug levels. It is also extremely important to follow these patients closely for potential adverse medication reactions.

Concentration-Dependent Killing of Aminoglycosides and Common Peaks and Troughs

Aminoglycosides are a class of drugs that have a very narrow therapeutic window and exhibit **concentration-dependent** bacterial killing. This means that aminoglycosides have the best bacterial killing potential when the concentration of the drug far exceeds the minimum inhibitory concentration (MIC) of the bacteria. Ideally, the peak should be 8–10 times greater than the MIC of the bacteria. Additionally, aminoglycosides are subject to a post-antibiotic effect. This post-antibiotic effect means that the bacteria will not benefit from additional doses of antibiotics for a period of time. Generally, a target aminoglycoside **peak** is 6–10 mcg/mL. The lowest effective peak should be used due to the potential of ototoxicity and nephrotoxicity. A target **trough** of below 1 mcg/mL is ideal.

Time-Dependent Killing of Vancomycin and Common Peaks and Troughs

Vancomycin is a drug that exhibits time-dependent bacterial killing and is generally only used in its intravenous form for gram positive cocci. Antibiotics that kill bacteria in a **time-dependent** fashion work best when antibiotic concentrations stay about the desired peak for as long as possible. It is best to dose vancomycin so that goal peaks are met and troughs do not drop to zero. Vancomycin is renally cleared and it is very important to renally dose this when needed. Generally, a target **vancomycin peak** is 10–30 mcg/mL. Higher troughs tend to have a higher incidence of adverse reactions such as neutropenia and potentially nephrotoxicity. As a general rule, only vancomycin peaks are measure and monitored. **Vancomycin troughs** can be monitored in critically ill and unstable patients.

Phase 1 and Phase 2 Biotransformation

Metabolism and biotransformation of drugs can be separated into two components: phase 1 and phase 2. During **phase 1 biotransformation**, a functional group such as a phenol group or amine group is either attached or uncovered on the main drug compound. **Phase 2 biotransformation** is also called phase 2 conjugation. During phase 2 biotransformation, functional groups such as glucuronic acid and other groups are added to the previously exposed functional group. The goal of this conjugation is to make the drug very polar. Polar drugs are in general easier to excrete renally as compared to electrically neutral drugs. Not all drugs undergo phase 1 and phase 2 biotransformation. Some drugs only undergo phase 2 biotransformation and some drugs do not undergo any biotransformation. These drugs are generally very polar in nature and are easily renally excreted.

Desensitization of Drug Receptors

Desensitization is also known as tolerance and may occur for numerous reasons. One reason is that a receptor becomes oversaturated by a ligand or drug. Receptors will become absorbed into the cells, in which the ligand is removed and the receptor is either degraded or returned to the cellular membrane. This process, which is necessary to recycle receptors that have become saturated, can lead to a down-regulation of drug activity and a down-regulation of therapeutic effects. Some drugs become tolerated faster than others. Morphine is a common drug that becomes well-tolerated or desensitized relatively quickly, and increased doses are needed to reach the same effect. Many tolerances toward a drug are generally reversible.

Physiologic Determinants of Pharmacokinetics

Physiologic determinants of pharmacokinetics include:

- **Cardiac output**: If low, this may delay the time of onset and also affect distribution as the resultant hypovolemia impairs blood flow to the tissues. Low cardiac output may also change the drug's half-life and concentrations in the plasma.
- **Pulmonary capacity**: Hypoxemia resulting from impaired pulmonary capacity may impair vascular, hepatic, and renal perfusion. Absorption of drugs may be delayed or incomplete and distribution decreased.
- **Celiac disease**: Drug absorption may vary depending on the drug with absorption decreased for some drugs (such as digoxin) and increased (such as aspirin and simvastatin) or delayed for others, affecting plasma concentrations.
- **Liver failure**: Because the liver is essential for the metabolism and elimination of many drugs, impaired liver function may increase plasma concentrations to toxic levels. Clearance of some drugs may be increased and others decreased. Protein-binding and distribution may be impaired for some drugs.
- **Pregnancy**: Gastric emptying and GI transit times are slowed, and this may affect drug absorption. Increased volume of plasma may affect protein binding. Increased levels of adipose tissue may increase distribution of lipid-soluble drugs. Hormone level increases and increased activity of enzymes may increase metabolism of some drugs resulting in lower active drug levels. Increased flow of blood to the kidneys and increased GFR may increase the rate of elimination of some drugs. Drug doses may need to be altered and some drugs discontinued because of teratogenic effect.
- **BMI**: Obesity, especially, is a concern because a high BMI may result in increased absorption of oral medications (because of increased rate of gastric emptying) but decreased absorption of subcutaneous drugs (because of added fatty tissue). Lipid-soluble drug distribution may increase and may accumulate in fatty tissue. Dosages of medications may need to be increased to reach the same effect. Protein binding may be affected. Reduced flow of blood to the liver may affect metabolism. Increased GFR may result in increased rate of drug elimination.

Race

While race is not a consideration with most medications, primarily because of a lack of research in how medications affect different ethnic populations, some racial groups respond differently from others to certain medications, and in some cases, a drug may be FDA-approved for only one ethnic group. For example, BiDil (a combination of isosorbide dinitrate and hydralazine), a medication for heart failure, is approved only for patients who self-identify as African Americans. (This does not mean it may be ineffective for others, only that it was tested on African Americans.) Drugs may be more or less readily absorbed by different races. Research indicates that African Americans respond less to beta blockers than to calcium channel blockers and better to multiple drugs than single therapy for hypertension. Asians and Hispanics tend to need lower doses of antipsychotic and antianxiety mediations and are at increased risk of toxic reactions from these drugs.

Influence of End-Stage Kidney Disease

Influence on Volume of Distribution of Various Drugs

End-stage kidney disease can drastically change the volume of **distribution** of many drugs. This change in volume of distribution can be due to variety of reasons including changes in drugs binding to various proteins, increased water weight gain, and other changes in the ratio of muscle to fat. In general, this change in volume of distribution will not affect the drug response to a large degree. For most medications, end-stage kidney disease increases the volume of distribution compared to a patient with normal kidney function. A few medications such as digoxin, pindolol, methicillin and ethambutol actually have a decreased volume of distribution compared to a patient with normal kidney function.

Influence on Protein Binding of Acidic Drugs

End-stage kidney disease can increase or decrease how much drug is **bound to proteins** in the body. Medications that are acidic, such as furosemide and phenytoin, generally are less protein bound. This decrease in protein binding can be caused by several factors including toxins binding to proteins, leading to less protein binding sites available for acidic drugs; changes in the amount of albumin in the body; and physical changes to protein binding sites. This is an important factor to keep in mind when checking kinetics for drugs such as phenytoin. If a patient has kidney dysfunction, they will likely have a greater amount of unbound phenytoin and therefore will be therapeutic in a lower target range.

Influence on Drug Metabolism

As a pharmacist, renally dosing medications is a common practice. It is important to understand that a patient with end-stage kidney disease not only has significantly reduced drug renal elimination, but also potentially metabolizes those drugs through altered pathways. Specifically, kidney disease has been shown to also alter how drugs are **metabolized** through the CYP P450 liver system. While this may not be the case for every patient with kidney disease, it is an important factor to consider if a patient is exhibiting signs of drug toxicity or is reacting differently to a medication than expected. If it does that metabolism of a drug is being affected, you will most likely need to reduce the dosage or frequency of the medication.

Pharmacogenomics

Pharmacogenomics

Pharmacogenomics is a generally new scientific field by which genomic techniques are used to measure differences in gene expression of individuals and populations, which might lead to a better understanding of drug response variability. By understanding the underlying regulation of drug metabolism in a given individual can allow for a more individualized therapeutic regimen. **Single nucleotide polymorphisms (SNP)**, are mutations, generally of a coding region of a gene, of a single nucleotide that occur at about a 5% frequency within the population. If these mutations do not change the overall protein sequence or protein function, it does not really matter; however, when these SNPs alter protein function, they can lead to small but significant changes in the phenotype, which can be important in the function and metabolism of a drug.

Genomics

Genomics is the field of study regarding the structure and function of the genome, an organism's set of DNA and genes. There are about 25,000 genes in a human, and each produces an average of 3 proteins. The DNA and genes are located on 23 pairs of chromosomes (22 pairs of autosomes and one pair of sex chromosomes) with each DNA strand comprised of 4 nucleotide bases: (A) adenine, (T) thymine, (G) guanine, and (C) cytosine with adenine always pairing with T (AT) and cytosine always pairing with G (CG). Genomics include sequencing (determining the correct order of the bases in DNA strands). The Human Genome Project (2003) provides the human genome sequence and is used as a reference for research into medical genomics. Researchers are now aware that one's genetic makeup has some effect on almost every disorder and are using genomics to better develop individualized medications and to understand response to medications.

Proteomics and Metabolomics

Proteomics (formed from *protein* and *genome*) is a study the proteomes, including the entire protein makeup of an organism, cell, or specific tissue under specified conditions because proteins changed in response to environmental influences. Proteins are generally identified through mass spectrometry and then organized utilizing bioinformatics. Proteases may be utilized to digest and help identify proteins. Proteomic studies are being done in research of diseases, such as cancer, heart disease, and psychiatric diseases. **Metabolomics** (formed from *metabolic* and *genome)* is the study of chemical processes that produce small-molecule metabolites in an organism, cell, or specific tissue (each has a distinct metabolic structure) providing information about its physiology and the products of its metabolism, usually through mass spectrometry. Metabolome changes in response to environmental factors, disease, and mutations, helping to identify disease states. The Human Metabolome Database has >40,000 entries regarding drugs, metabolites, and hormones identified in the human body.

Pharmacists' Role in Pharmacogenetics/Pharmacogenomics

Pharmacists will play an important role in pharmacogenetics/pharmacogenomics. Pharmacists can have important roles in researching the effect of important single nucleotide polymorphisms (SNPs) which can regulate drug activity in a certain subset of the population. Pharmacists can have important roles in reading genetic tests, individualizing treatments based on the patients' genetic makeup, counseling people about their particular genetic polymorphisms so that the patient can understand more about their own healthcare issues. For this will need a better understanding of pharmacogenomics in order to be strong leaders in healthcare in the not so distant future.

Genetic Drift

Genetic drift is the chance that an allele will mutate, leading to various changes in biological traits but generally does not alter the entire genetics of the population, does not offer any adaptation, and thus is technically separate from natural selection, although the two processes often occur simultaneously. Genetic drift is a common reason for small genetic differences between people and population subsets, such as polymorphisms. Genetic drift also occurs in viruses and other microbial agents, such as influenza, which is important in the variability of the virus that is observed throughout the world and why it is difficult to create an effective vaccine.

Linkage Disequilibrium

Linkage disequilibrium is a term used in genetics to describe the association of alleles at two different loci (fixed genetic position of a chromosome) often on different chromosomes. Linkage disequilibrium is used in population genetics to measure the frequency of haplotype formation and genetic changes which deviates from the frequency if mutations were simply random. It is thought that this process is evolutionarily conserved, allowing for greater genetic variability within a population, and also leads to the formation of SNPs. Many factors can regulate linkage disequilibrium including natural selection, genetic drift, gene conversion, rates of genetic recombination, as well as rates of mutation.

SNPs That Alter Metabolism of Codeine and BiDil

A small subset of the Caucasian population has a mutation in the **CYP2D6 enzyme**. CYP2D6 is an important metabolic enzyme. It has roles in metabolizing the opioid drug codeine. To be effective, codeine must be metabolized into morphine. People lacking a proper functioning CYP2D6 enzyme, cannot metabolize the drug into morphine, thus codeine has no effect. Another example of population differences in relationship to drug therapies include isosorbide dinitrate and hydralazine (BiDil) was a drug that was originally denied by the FDA because it didn't show an effective treatment against heart disease in the general population, but in later tests showed a significant effect in a subset of the African American population. The genetic basis for this drug therapy has not been fully elucidated.

Effects of the SNP of Thiopurine Methyltransferase

A relatively common SNP causes a defect in the **thiopurine methyltransferase (TMPT)**. The enzyme is important in methylation of thiopurine compounds. It also has important roles in regulating chemotherapy drugs such as 6-methylcaptoporurine, azathioprine, and 6-thioguanine, all of which have important immunosuppressive qualities. People with a mutated TMPT often cannot metabolize these drugs properly which can often lead to severe adverse reactions such as severe bone marrow toxicity, which occurs when bone marrow is severely depressed. This suppression of the bone marrow allows for acute infections to take hold and possibly be fatal to the patient. New tests are now available for TMPT defects. It is presently used to titer doses for individual people. People without the defect get the normal dose of the immunosuppressants, while people with the defect will get a much lower dose and still show therapeutic effects.

Diminished Metabolizers and Ultra-Metabolizers

Often times SNPs will cause one of two types of changes in drug metabolizing; these include **diminished metabolizers** and **ultra-metabolizers.** Diminished metabolizers, often caused by mutations in the metabolic pathway which generally leads to increased bioavailability of the drug, increased drug activity, and increased toxicity if the patient took an active compound. If a poor-metabolizer took a pro-drug however, this could lead to a diminished response and decreased bioavailability. Ultra-metabolizers have increased levels of metabolism, which can lead to a decreased bioavailability, and decreased effectiveness of the drug if the patient took an active drug. If they are taking a pro-drug, however, this could increase the bioavailability of the active component and lead to a toxic response.

Polymorphisms of MDR1, 2AR, and SUR

Almost a quarter of the population has a SNP in the **multi-drug resistance gene 1 (MDR1)**, a drug transporter, which can lead to an increased amount of plasma levels of Digoxin, which can lead to increased bioavailability and increased toxicity of the drug. Over one quarter of the population has a SNP in the **Beta-2 adrenergic (2AR)** receptors which can weaken the response of beta-2 agonists such as Albuterol. A rare subset of the population has a SNP in the **Sulphonylurea receptor gene (SUR)** which can lead to decreased insulin response and can decrease the activity of Tolbutamide.

Major Challenges of Pharmacogenetic Testing

Pharmacogenetic testing can be very difficult and overwhelming to perform, particularly since the amount of information out there is immense. Ideally it would be nice to be able to test the complete genome for any possible SNPs, receiving a complete view of every individual's genetic makeup in order to efficiently and effectively individualize therapy. However, in reality, this is not feasible, as it would take a massive amount of time and resources to do this. In reality it would be more feasible to test particular gene SNPs, thus keeping the pharmacogenetic tests manageable. This could unfortunately lead to the neglect of other prominent SNPs. It is also important to understand and study the mechanistic relationship between genotype and phenotype further. An understanding of the link between observed genetic SNPs and mutated phenotypes is necessary before truly effective testing can be performed. This type of testing is important, however, and even as limited as it is now, it can save countless lives.

Gender Differences in Drug Metabolism

There is increasing evidence that **gender** differences exist in relationship to drug metabolism, although these differences are not entirely understood. Certain drugs for example have faster metabolism in the different sexes. Propranolol was metabolized at a rate 50% faster in men than in women through oxidative metabolism. Other drugs such as chlordiazepoxide and lidocaine are also metabolized faster in men than women. Other drugs are metabolized faster in women than men such as caffeine, diazepam, and acetaminophen. These differences can be in part due to differences in phase I and phase II metabolism, such as differences in oxidation reactions and cytochrome p450 enzymes.

Glucose 6-Phosphate Dehydrogenase Deficiencies

Deficiencies can occur in glucose 6-phosphate dehydrogenase which can lead to several blood problems such as hemolytic anemia. Historically this disorder has gone seemingly unnoticed until the ingestion of uncooked fava beans, which causes the victim to fall very ill. Blood cells which show a sharp decline in 6-phosphate dehydrogenase undergo hemolysis in response to uncooked fava beans as well as a few particular drugs. The exact mechanism is not well understood. People with this deficiency should not be given anti- malarial drugs, sulfonamides, nitrofurans, acetaminophen, acetylsalicylic acid or vitamin K. This deficiency is more common in males, as it is an X-linked sex trait; however, homozygous females are somewhat common in comparison to other sex linked disorders.

Effects of Polymorphisms of UDP Glucuronosyltransferase SNPs

UDP glucuronosyltransferase (UGT) 1A6 is an important component of the glucuronidation metabolism pathways found in the liver. Glucuronidation metabolism is important in the detoxification of phase I drug metabolites. **Polymorphisms of the UGT1A6 gene** can have major effects on drug metabolism. It has been shown that UGT1A6 can lead to problems in metabolism of phenolic drugs. Heterozygous UGT1A6 SNPs have moderate decreased activity of many drugs, due to increased metabolism. People who possess homozygous SNPs of UGT1A6 have a higher level of glucuronidation and decreased activity of many drugs including acetaminophen, morphine, beta-blockers, and cyclosporine A. SNPs in UGT1A1 were shown to lead to increased adverse drug reactions in relationship to irinotecan. Additionally, UGT1A1 SNPs have been connected to disorders including Gilbert's syndrome and Crigler-Najjar Syndrome. Gilbert's Syndrome is a heritable disease that leads to chronic decreased metabolism of bilirubin, leading to a mild decrease in clearance of the protein. Crigler-Najjar Syndrome is a more severe disease involved in decreased bilirubin metabolism, which is chronic and can be fatal if untreated.

Effects of N-Acetyltransferase Polymorphisms

There are two forms of N-acetyltransferase (NAT1 and NAT2), both of which can have important polymorphisms. N-acetyltransferase has important roles in metabolism, which transfers the acetyl groups to arylamine compounds. Acetylation is an important step in both synthesis and breakdown of numerous biological components. More is known however about the clinical relevance of **NAT2 polymorphisms**. NAT2 polymorphisms can lead to adverse drug reactions to such drugs as isoniazid, hydralazine, procainamide, sulphasalazine. People administered with isoniazid who have a NAT2 polymorphism suffer from peripheral neuropathy. Other adverse reactions include lupus erythematosus with administration of hydralazine or procainamide and hemolysis in response to sulphasalazine.

Extemporaneous Compounding

ASHP Guidelines on Safe Handling of Hazardous Drugs

American Society of Health-System Pharmacists (**ASHP**) guidelines on **safe handling of hazardous drugs** includes:

- Policies and a safety program must be in place for all circumstances in which hazardous drugs are handles, and all such drugs must be labeled as requiring safe handling procedures.
- Safe drug handling policies must cover receiving, storing and transporting. All storage packages and areas must be properly labeled and provide adequate safety of substances/drugs contained. Transporting must be done in such a manner as to reduce environmental contamination with breakage.
- Hazardous drugs must be handled in designated areas and only compounded and administered by individuals trained to handle hazardous drugs.
- Engineering controls and C-PECS (ventilated device) must be in place to protect workers in C-SECS (outside vented or physically-separated room). Containment supplemental engineering devices, such as the closed-system drug-transfer device, must be utilized.
- PPE must be appropriate for hazardous materials. Disposable PPE must not be reused and non-disposable PPE (face guards) must be properly decontaminated. Double-gloves are recommended for drug handling.
- Hazardous drugs are disposed of as hazardous waste and must follow state and EPA regulations, and medical screening and environmental sampling should be done.

NIOSH Guidelines on Safe Handling of Hazardous Drugs

NIOSH divided hazardous drugs into 3 groups because safety requirements may vary:

1. Antineoplastic drugs, many pose reproductive risk.
2. Non-antineoplastic drugs, some pose reproductive risk.
3. Pose risks primarily to men/women actively trying to conceive and pregnant or breast-feeding women.

Safe handling recommendations include:

- Routinely assess hazards before handling hazardous drugs, review current inventory, and conduct regular training.
- Establish program for safe handling of hazardous drugs, including proper use and maintenance of equipment. The program must cover receiving and storing drugs (handle spills, labeling, PPE, store hazardous drug separately), drug preparation (ventilated cabinet, PPE with double gloves, closed system transfer devices), administration (use protective medical devices, PPE, safe tubing handling, double-bagging), ventilated cabinets (use to mix prepare, or handle hazardous drugs), air flow and exhaust (use HEPA filters for exhaust and have outside exhaust), maintenance (establish protocols), routine cleaning and contamination (do before and after each activity/work shift), housekeeping (use appropriate PPE), waste disposal (place contaminated items and sharps in yellow-chemotherapy waste containers), spill control (follow written policies/procedures), and medical surveillance (follow OSHA guidelines).

FDA's Regulation of Compounding

Compounded drugs are not FDA approved, but in response to infections and deaths from contaminated drugs, the Drug Quality and Security Act (DOSA) (2013) was passed and updated the Federal Food, Drug, and Cosmetic Act related to drug compounding, Section 503a. Compounding is generally regulated by state boards of pharmacy under FDA guidance in compliance with the DF&C Act. FDA guidelines include conditions under which pharmacists and physicians are exempt from requirements of provisions usually applied to drugs (good manufacturing process, labeling, and new drug applications). Compounded drugs must be compounded for individual patients by licensed pharmacists/physicians with approved bulk drug substances or drug products. Compounders should avoid providing large amounts of drugs that are essentially copies of commercially available drugs.

Regulatory requirements include:

- No dirty or contaminated products may be used in the compound.
- If the compound claims to equal a drug, it must meet the same standards and have the same strength.
- Labeling must be correct with no false or misleading information and must contain adequate directions for use.
- Unapproved new drugs may not be compounded.

USP Standards

The **United States Pharmacopeia** outlines quality and safety standards for medications and pharmacies. Those relevant to the pharmacy include general chapters 795, 797, and 800:

- **USP General Chapter 795 Pharmaceutical Compounding: Nonsterile Preparations** focuses on applying good compounding practices to the process of preparing nonsterile compounded medications. This includes, but is not limited to, the compounding process, facility requirements, personnel training, documentation, and quality controls.

- **USP General Chapter 797 Pharmaceutical Compounding: Sterile Preparations** provides the procedures and requirements for compounding sterile medications. This includes, but is not limited to, training and responsibilities of compounding personnel, environmental monitoring and controls, storage and testing of finished preparations, and infection control methods. USP 797 covers compounding standards for non-hazardous and hazardous sterile products.
- **USP General Chapter 800 Hazardous Drugs: Handling in Healthcare Settings** focuses on standards for the safe handling of hazardous drugs in healthcare settings to minimize the risk of exposure to personnel, patients, and the environment.

Important Guidelines of Quality Compounding Including Beyond-Use-Dates

There are important **quality control guidelines that should be followed when compounding.** These guidelines include maintaining the utmost care when compounding any drug and not cutting any corners. It important to maintain accurate measurements, processing procedures, packaging, record-keeping and properly assigned beyond-use-dates. Beyond-use-dates are expiration dates assigned by the pharmacist that are based on drug degradation. A pharmacist, when deciding on a beyond-use-date, needs to strike a balance long enough for the drug to be used by the patient according to the dosing regimen on the prescription, but not too long that the drug will degrade and become useless for therapeutic treatment.

Shelf-Life

Drugs have a finite period of time before they degrade and are no longer effective therapeutically. This period of time, which begins as soon as the drug is manufactured and stored, is known as the shelf-life of a drug, is the period of time by which a drug from the moment it is manufactured will. **Shelf-life** of a drug or dosage form of a drug can be determined by using the Arrhenius equation: log (k2/k1) = (Ea (T2-T1))/2.303RT2T1. k2 and k1 are the rates of the reaction at the absolute temperatures which are described as T2 & T1. R= the gas constant. Ea is the activation energy of the experiment. This reaction can give a best estimate of the amount of time that a drug will be effective before full degradation occurs.

Tablets

A tablet is a solid formulation of a drug made for the purpose of easier storage and administration. Effervescence tablets are dissolved in water before they are taken. Effervescence occurs when carbon dioxide is released through the reaction of sodium bicarbonate in water, which helps dissolve the tablet and release the drug into the solution. Chewable tablets are used for a more rapid absorption of a drug. The drug is released through chewing and interaction with saliva. Buccal and sublingual tablets are dissolved in the presence of saliva. These type of drugs are preferred if avoidance of the first-pass effect is desired. Time release tablets can also be called sustained released tablets, which are formulations that have several doses of a drug, though each dose is not released into the system until a certain time has passed. They can potentially reduce adverse reactions and improve adherence of a drug. Coated tablets are created to improve taste and to prevent premature dissolving once swallowed. Enteric-coated drugs for example resist the stomach acids and dissolve in the intestines.

Agents Used in Tablet Formulation

A tablet is a mixture of a drug and inactive carrier/ ingredients that is formulated into a solid, generally for easy oral consumption and absorption into the body, often through the gastrointestinal tract. Tablets are **formulated with various** agents including diluents, adsorbents, moistening agents, binding agents, glidants, lubricants and disintegrating agents. Diluent agents are also known as bulking agents such as sucrose of NaCl, which is used with low-dose drugs to bring the weight of the tablet to at least 50 mg, for easier handling and use. Adsorbents are agents that can bind and sequester fluids keeping them dry, in granules before being compressed into a tablet. Absorbents include silica. Moistening agents are used to keep compounds during a wet granulation process. Moistening agents include water and isopropanol. Binding agents are used to adhere moist granulations during tablet formation. Binding agents include starch, cellulose, and polyvinylpyrrolidone. Glidants are compounds use to improve friction and flow of granulated components of a tablet. Glidants include silica, starch and talc powder. Lubricants are also used, mainly during the manufacturing process so that the tablets do not stick or remain in the manufacturing machines, thus the tablets do not break.

Emulsions

An emulsion consists of at least two liquids that will not mix with each other such as oil and water. Instead, one of the liquid phases (dispersed phase) (i.e. oil) will be diffused throughout the second liquid phase (continuous phase) (i.e. water) as droplets or globules. This mixture is stabilized by emulsifying agents. The two most common types of emulsions are oil-in water (o/w) or water-in-oil (w/o). O/w emulsions generally have oil globules dissolved into an aqueous phase. W/o emulsions have water globules dissolved into an oil phase. Emulsions are often used as lotions, ointments and creams. Common o/w emulsifying agents include sodium lauryl sulfate, sodium oleate and glyceryl monostearate. Common w/o emulsifying agents include calcium palmitate, sorbitan esters, cholesterol and wool fat products.

Unstable Emulsions

Emulsions can become **unstable** by creaming and sedimentation, breaking, coalescence, aggregation, phase inversion and through microorganism growth. Creaming occurs in response to an upward movement of particles (globules) in the dispersed phase in relation to the continuous phase. (i.e. oil droplets moving upward through the aqueous phase). Sedimentation is the opposite of creaming, when the particles are globules move downward through the continuous phase. Both are reversible by remixing the emulsion compound but can lead to other problems in emulsion instability. If during sedimentation or creaming, the protective film that surrounds the dispersed globules breaks, this can lead to breaking of the emulsion, causing the globules to coalesce into larger globular particles or aggregate into larger clumps. Phase inversion occurs when an emulsion goes from a w/o emulsion to an o/w emulsion or o/w emulsion to a w/o emulsion. Changes in electrolytes and the addition of different emulsifying agents can lead to this effect. Also, microorganisms can grow on emulsion destroying emulsifying agents. Preservatives are usually added to prevent such a thing to occur.

Commonly Used Solutions

Solutions are homogenous mixtures of one or more substances in a solvent such as water. There are different types of solutions, including syrups, elixirs, and tinctures.

- A **syrup** consists of sugar, usually sucrose, or other flavoring agents dissolved in water along with the drug of choice.
- An **elixir** consists of a sweetened solution of water and ethanol, along with the drug or drugs of choice.
- A **spirit** is generally considered a solution of alcohol and water that is mixed with volatile and pungent compounds and drugs.
- **Tinctures** are generally vegetable based extracts formed in either alcohol or alcohol/water solutions.

Solutions are often taken orally. If kept sterile, solutions can also be used for injectable drugs such as antibiotics, pain medication, etc.

Type A Prescription Balances

Type A (type III) prescription balances are an important component of a compounding pharmacy and are used to accurately weigh and measure reagents in order to create a functional and safe therapeutic drug. Accuracy of a type A prescription balance must be kept in good working condition, and its sensitivity and accuracy should be determined periodically. The United States Pharmacopeia (USP) regulates four specific tests to determine the sensitivity of the balance: the sensitivity determination test, the arm-ratio test, shift test and the rider graduate-beam test. The sensitivity determination test requires a 6 mg weight to determine the sensitivity of the balance up to a 6 mg. The arm-ratio test is used to detect inaccuracies between the lengths of the arms of the balance. The shift test is used to determine if the arms and the levels of the balance have been shifted out of place, a good test to determine misuse of the balance. The graduate-beam test is used to measure inaccuracies of the weigh-beam and rider of the balance.

HEPA Filters

HEPA stands for **High Efficiency Particulate Air filter** or **High Efficiency Particulate Arresting filter.** It is an air filter that is important in compounding hoods to maintain sterility of the drugs and other compounding reagents needed to compound the drug. The HEPA filter acts as a blockade, made up of meshed fibers spaced no more than 3 μm apart, thus removing anything larger than 3 μm. Additionally, other smaller compounds will often stick to the meshed fibers, rather than crossing through the filter. Using a fast airstream across the filter can greatly decrease the diffusion rate of particulates in the air, to an area of 0.1 μm, easily inhibiting bacterial and viral contamination. Efficiency of HEPA filters should be tested often and replaced when efficiency drops in order to maintain the integrity of the compounding pharmacy.

Extemporaneous Dispensing

Extemporaneous dispensing or compounding is the process of mixing together different ingredients to make an unlicensed prescription or drug formula. This is a high-risk procedure because steps must be carried out with care to avoid error, exposure to hazardous chemicals, or contamination of ingredients. Extemporaneous dispensing may be utilized if the desired dosage is unavailable, a drug or specific formula is unavailable, or the form of the drug (tablet) must be changed (to liquid, for example). Sometimes, adult medications are dispensed extemporaneously in liquid form for pediatric patients. Active ingredients are generally obtained from available commercial medications or from chemicals. Extemporaneous dispensing should be done only if a commercial product is unavailable. The pharmacist should review data regarding drug stability and solution kinetics (for liquids), should not assign extemporaneous dispensing to unlicensed assistants, and should ensure that the ingredients and ultimate dosage are correct and that the label provides adequate information. Alternatives, such as cutting scored tablets or administering a drug by a different route, should be explored.

Tests to Measure Laminar Flow Efficiency

The following are tests that measure laminar flow efficiency:

- **Smoke test**: By creating a "smoky" atmosphere. This can be performed a number of ways, including putting dry ice in water, and observing the dissipation of "smoke" in the laminar hood, to measure airflow, to determine that the hood is working properly.
- **DOP Test**: Using aerosol DiOctyl Phthalate (DOP). The DOP test can be used to measure particulate penetration of the HEPA filter in the laminar hood.

- **Microbial Test**: With the use of a device known as a microbial sampler, can be used to sample air quality of the laminar hood to measure levels of microorganisms and can also be used to measure other levels of possible contaminates.

Sterilization Techniques

Sterilization techniques are as follows:

- **Filtration**: Uses a filter with a certain pore size such as .2 micron, in which anything above .2 microns will not go through the filter. Generally, compounded products should be filter sterilized with a .2 micron filter; however, to avoid clogging of the filter, a larger pore size should be used first to remove bigger particles. Two types of filters are generally used, hydrophilic filters for aqueous solutions and hydrophobic filters for gases and volatile solvents.
- **Heat sterilization** is another technique used by compounding pharmacies and research labs. **Autoclaving** uses a mixture of heat, moisture and pressure to kill microbial agents and sterilize solutions and labware. It is usually quick, yet very effective.
- **Dry sterilization** uses an oven at very high temperatures and filtered air to sterilize products. Dry sterilization uses hotter temperatures for longer periods of time than an autoclave. Used to remove impurities (pyrogens) from lab and compounding equipment.
- **Ethanol Sterilization**: 70% ethanol is considered to be the most effective concentration of ethanol for sterilization techniques. A greater percentage of ethanol does not provide greater sterilization, and thus, it is more cost-effective to use 70% ethanol. Ethanol kills bacteria and other organisms by denaturing proteins and disrupting the cell wall/cell membrane of cells. Additionally, it is thought that 95% - 100% ethanol evaporates so rapidly that it does not have a chance to fully kill bacteria and other microbes.
- **Ultraviolet (UV) Sterilization**: Many hoods are connected with ultraviolet lights which are used for sterilization. At a wavelength of approximately 250 nm, the UV light can lead to DNA breaks which can lead to thymine dimers in DNA, inhibiting replication, transcription and translation of the microbial organisms, leading to the death of the microbial cells.

Important Terms

Admixture: IV drugs that are sterilely combined together in one IV bag before administration.

Aseptic Technique: Performing procedures in a sterile environment to minimize contamination.

Controlled Area (Buffer Area): The area where the laminar flow workbench is located in the pharmacy. This area should remain as clean as possible to reduce contamination chances.

Critical Site: Any space that can lead to a possible contamination between a sterile product and the outside environment. Must be tightly controlled and regulated.

Hypertonic: Solution that has higher levels of solutes than red blood cells, which will lead to shrinking of the cells.

Hypotonic: Opposite to hypertonic, can lead to bursting of red blood cells.

Isotonic: Solutions that are similar to body fluids, similar osmotic and diffusive pressures which should not lead to stress on red blood cells and other cell types.

Poison: Everything is a poison. A poison simply depends on the dose and level used to lead to a toxic response, an injury to a tissue or organism as a whole. Water is essential for life; however, too much of it can be quite toxic to living cells. On the other hand, something that is a known poison might have therapeutic effects. For example anti-cancer drugs are highly toxic; however, at certain doses and drug regimens, they can be used to kill cancers.

Toxin: Any toxic agent that is produced by a biological system (plant, fungi, animal, or microbe) such as rattle snake poison, or botulism toxin.

Toxicant: Any toxic agent that has been created due to some natural or human endeavors but do not have a biological basis. Nerve gases like ricin or other toxic agents such as dioxin or arsenic are examples of toxicants

Social/Behavioral/Administrative Sciences

Pharmacy Law and Regulatory Affairs

HIPAA

In hospital and retail pharmacies, patient privacy is of the utmost importance. Pharmacy management must ensure that prescription and medical records of individual patients remain private. The **Health Insurance Portability and Accountability Act (HIPAA)** was passed in 1996 and makes it easier for patients to obtain their own protected health information (PHI, medical records), but harder for other non-authorized people to do so. To maintain confidentiality of PHI, a pharmacy must adopt several regulations, including when speaking to a patient about their prescriptions, do their best to keep their voices low, have a specific semi-private or private counseling area, or ask other customers to wait a few feet back until they are done with their present patient. Additionally it is a good idea to secure computer access to keep PHI safe, remind employees to logout of the computer before walking away, and only allow people who need to see the PHI to do certain tasks for the patient (i.e. fill prescriptions, talk to the insurance company, counsel patients or talk to physicians about the patient).

Classifications of Controlled Substances

Classifications of controlled substances are as follows:

- **Class I:** Drugs with this classification are often abused and highly addictive but are not considered therapeutically useful. These drugs include recreational drugs such as heroine and methamphetamines.
- **Class II**: Drugs that have a propensity for abuse and addiction but have use in medical treatment. These include opioids such as morphine and oxycontin.
- **Class III**: Drugs have a propensity for abuse and addiction but less than previous classifications and have a therapeutic uses. Drugs of this class include vicodin and hydrocodone.
- **Class IV**: Propensity of abuse still exists, though less than previous classes. This class includes drugs such as soma, midrin and valium.
- **Class V**: Includes over-the-counter medications which are considered low propensity for abuse or addiction, such as ibuprofen (Advil®), acetaminophen (Tylenol®) and diphenhydramine (Benadryl®).

Anti-Tampering Act of 1982 and Federal Law of Medicinal Use of Alcohol

After a slew of post-retail contaminations occurred with cyanide in Tylenol leading to several deaths, the **Anti-Tampering Act of 1982** was passed that makes it a federal offense to tamper with consumer products. From this act more stringent tamper-proof and quality control mechanisms were developed to stop such a tragedy from occurring again. The **Federal Law of Medicinal Use of Alcohol** states that if alcohol being sold is only used for medicinal purposes, a federal medicinal spirits dealer's stamp is required, rather than an alcohol license from the US Bureau of Alcohol, Tobacco, and Firearms, which is required for alcohol sold for any other purposes.

Pure Food and Drug Act and the Food, Drug, and Cosmetic Act

The **Pure Food and Drug Act** was passed in 1906 and gave the federal government the power to regulate and inspect all food and drug products for safety, and made it a federal crime to sell food that had been tampered with or poisoned. Additionally, this act enforced the proper labeling of foods. This act paved way for the eventual creation of the Food and Drug Administration. The **Food, Drug, and Cosmetic Act** was passed in 1938 after several deaths in children occurred in response to a normally safe drug, sulfanilamide, being dissolved into a rather toxic substance, diethylene glycol, before being sold to consumers. This prompted the government to take action and, among other things, provided authority to regulate the safety of food, drugs and cosmetics.

Durham-Humphrey Amendment of 1951 and the Kefauver Harris Amendment of 1962

The **Durham-Humphrey Amendment** was passed in 1951 in order to regulate potentially addictive and harmful drugs. It states that these drugs must only be sold to a licensed practitioner such as a doctor who must prescribe the drugs to the patients. After this act was passed, certain drugs could no longer be purchased by the patient directly from the manufacturer, but instead must be purchased only after a legal prescription for the drug has be written for them. The **Kefauver Harris Amendment** was passed in 1962 after the marketed drug thalidomide was shown to cause severe fetal disorders. This amendment proposed that a drug must be safe and show efficacy (activity against a desired disease state) before it would be approved for marketing. Additionally, the burden of proof for the safety and efficacy of a drug now lied solely on the manufacturer. If it could not show reasonable cost-benefit effect, a drug would not be approved for market.

Medical Device Amendment Act of 1976

An amendment to the **Federal Food and Drug Cosmetic Act** that created classes of regulation for medical devices depening on the activity and safety of the medical devices.

- **Class I devices** require the least amounts of controls before they are sold and used, are considered to have limited possibility for causing harm, and are also simple in design and use.
- **Class II devices** are when controls used for class I devices are insufficient and other standardized controls are needed before the devices are allowed to reach the market and used by patients.
- **Class III devices** consist of most medical devices; they need approval by the FDA before reaching the market. These devices are generally those that are needed to save or sustain human life and health.

Drugs Exempt from the Poison Prevention Act

The **Poison Prevention Act** put into place the use of safety caps on medicine. Some drugs, however, are exempt from this law. These include nitroglycerine, isosorbide dinitrate at a dose less than 10 mg, cholestyrmine, methylprednisolone, mebendazole, potassium dietary supplements, oral contraceptives, erythromycin, ethyl succinate, colestipol, pancrelipase, and prednisone. Some other regulations might be required like certain doses and dosage forms which make certain drugs exempt from this law.

Prescription Drug User Fee Act and the FDA Modernization Act

The **Drug User Fee Act (PDUFA)** was passed in 1992, which gave the FDA the power to charge the pharmaceutical manufacturers a fee, which can be used to increase the drug review. This law was passed to improve and modernize the drug review process. However, this act only allowed fees to be charged until 1997. The **FDA Modernization act (FDMA)** was passed in 1997, which increased the time period by which the FDA could charge drug manufacturers a fee until 2002. This act allowed the FDA to increase the drug review process, as well as to decrease the review time of potentially lifesaving drugs, allowing them to reach the market faster. This ability however, has its controversy, allowing sometimes-unsafe drugs to reach the market.

Orphan Drug Act of 1983 and OBRA Act of 1990

The **Orphan Drug Act of 1983** encourages pharmaceutical companies to develop and produce drugs for rare diseases that may only affect a small percentage of patients in relation to the population as a whole. These drugs are known as orphan drugs. This law provides tax breaks and other incentives for pharmaceutical companies for creating these generally non-profitable drugs. The **OBRA Act** was passed in 1990 and proposes that pharmacists must properly counsel patients on new prescriptions, making sure that the patients understand the instructions that are needed to take this new drug therapy. This is very important to decrease toxicity and increase effectiveness of the prescription.

Main Components OBRA '90

Omnibus Budget Reconciliation Act of 1990 (OBRA '90) has a few main components that address pharmacy regulations. The components include regular and proper drug utilization reviews (DUR's), collecting data on drug safety and efficacy, and patient counseling. The first main goal of OBRA '90 relates to improving drug therapy and medication safety through the DUR's and proper drug interaction reviews. The second main goal of OBRA '90 relates to patient counseling. According to OBRA '90, proper patient counseling must be given to patients when a new prescription is dispensed. Patient medication counseling includes items such as proper administration of medications and possible medication, diet and herbal drug interactions.

OBRA '90 in Relation to Patient Medication Counseling

The OBRA '90 act proposed new **federal laws requiring pharmacists to counsel on new prescriptions and new refills**. Each state has its own requirements as well. It is good for pharmacists to familiarize themselves with federal laws as well as counseling laws from the states they wish to be licensed. OBRA '90 proposes that a pharmacist will need to discuss various counseling points: the name of the drug, description of the drug, special instructions for the administration of the drug, possible adverse reactions, possible interactions and contraindications, as well as how many refills are left on the prescription and directions in case a dose of the medicine is missed.

OSHA

OSHA (**Occupational Safety and Health Administration**) is an agency that falls under the control of the US Department of Labor in response to the congressional law, the Occupational Safety and Health Act. OSHA provides important regulations for work place environments to insure a safe, healthy working environment. OSHA regulates the need for gloves, respirators and various other protective gear and clothing to reduce exposures of possible dangerous chemicals with which an employee might come into contact. These protective gears, as regulated by OSHA, are known as personal protective equipment (PPE). Other important OSHA regulations include permissible exposure levels (PELs) to dangerous chemicals which must be kept at a minimum. Other important requirements that regulate everything from eye strain to muscle aches are controlled by OSHA. If a business fails to follow OSHA guidelines, they can be held liable and suffer severe fines and possible lawsuits from injured employees.

Review Video: Intro to OSHA
Visit mometrix.com/academy and enter code: 913559

DEA

The **Drug Enforcement Agency**'s job is to enforce the controlled substance act that was passed in 1970 and it shares jurisdiction with the FBI, involving of selling, smuggling, and abuse of illegal narcotics in the United States. The DEA has important authority in designating who can prescribe federally controlled therapeutic drugs and what federally controlled therapeutic drugs can be prescribed.

DEA Number

Healthcare practitioners, as well as healthcare institutions that have prescriptive authority, must register with the DEA and receive a DEA number. The **DEA number** provides federally regulated prescriptive authority and tracks the use of controlled substances. The DEA number is made up of 2 letters, six numbers, and a checksum digit. The first letter is the letter that designates the type of registrant (i.e. practitioner versus a clinic); the second letter is the last initial of the registrant's surname. The seventh digit is known as a checksum digit and is used to test the validity of the DEA number. By adding the second, fourth and sixth numbers and multiplying this sum by two, then adding the first, third and fifth numbers, then taking these two numbers and adding them together, the last digit of this answer is the checksum digit of the DEA number. If this mathematical equation does not work with a DEA number, the DEA number is not valid.

Exceptions to Informed Consent

There are times that **exceptions to informed consent** can occur. When these exceptions occur, details of healthcare do not need to be addressed to patients. These exceptions occur during:

- Public health emergencies (e.g., outbreak of a disease when quarantine is needed).
- Medical emergencies (in matters of life and death it is not necessary particularly if the patient is incapacitated).
- Incompetency (a patient is unable to make a correct informed decision. This is controversial and often times a court order is needed to deem someone as incompetent).
- The patient waives the right to informed consent, which could be for any number of reasons such as cultural or religious, but this waiver and retracted at any time by the patient.

Liability of Pharmacist in Relation to Medical Errors

A pharmacist is held **liable** for prescription mistakes, especially if injuries are caused by apparent negligence. Additionally, the pharmacy and pharmacists can be held liable for mistakes that are made by people working for them, including interns and technicians. Additionally the pharmacy will be held liable as well. Although malpractice insurance will cover some costs, the insurance premiums can be excessive. It is important to decrease errors as much as possible in a pharmacy and keep a close eye on technicians and interns. Be firm about mistakes to decrease the liability, but also understand mistakes happen. Fix any as soon as possible and always be courteous.

Ethical Decision Making

Principles of Biomedical Ethics

Beneficence and Nonmaleficence

Beneficence is an ethical principle that involves performing actions that are for the purpose of benefitting another person. In the care of a patient, any procedure or treatment should be done with the ultimate goal of benefitting the patient, and any actions that are not beneficial should be reconsidered. As a patient's condition changes, procedures need to be continually reevaluated to determine if they are still of benefit. **Nonmaleficence** is an ethical principle that means healthcare workers should provide care in a manner that does not cause direct intentional harm to the patient:

- The actual act must be good or morally neutral.
- The intent must be only for a good effect.
- A bad effect cannot serve as the means to get to a good effect.
- A good effect must have more benefit than a bad effect has harm.

Autonomy and Justice

Autonomy is the ethical principle that the individual has the right to make decisions about his or her own care. In the case of children, the child cannot make autonomous decisions, so the parents serve as the legal decision maker. The pharmacist must keep patients fully informed so that they can exercise their autonomy in informed decision-making. **Justice** is the ethical principle that relates to the distribution of the limited resources of healthcare benefits to the members of society. These resources must be distributed fairly. This issue may arise if there is only one bed left and two patients. Justice comes into play in deciding which patient should stay and which should be transported or otherwise cared for. The decision should be made according to what is best or most just for the patients and not colored by personal bias.

Ethical Situations Pharmacists May Encounter

One big **ethical issue** that pharmacists will need to face when dealing with patients or dealing with fellow pharmacists, is the issue of morals and dispensing of prescriptions and other drugs. So as a pharmacist you must ask yourself if your personal beliefs are more important than that of the health of a patient. This is a major controversy in the realm of pharmacy and healthcare, because many believe that it is not the right of pharmacists or physicians to "choose" who they treat or not treat. However, many healthcare personnel do not believe they should have to do something that they are morally against. There is no correct choice, but there are important choices that need to be made nonetheless. One example could be selling needles to drug addicts; on one hand this might be construed as propagating illegal narcotic use, however, it can be also be a means to decrease the possible exchange of dangerous infectious diseases such as HIV and hepatitis.

Ethical Issue of Pharmaceutics During Drug Development

Pharmaceutical companies develop and screen new drugs for various disease states, and for any that show promise, the companies will patent them immediately. The patent allows protection for approximately seventeen years on a drug. However, it will take eleven of those years for this patented compound to reach the market. The compound must go through pre-clinical and clinical trials to show safety and efficacy in a human population, before the FDA will approve it. The problem lies in that this only gives the pharmaceutical companies a seven-year window to make a profit over the 800 million dollars spent in the development of the drug, if the compound passes all the requirements. This type of process builds an intense pressure to get drugs to market, which could lead to relatively unsafe drugs reaching the market with unforeseen toxicities. The pharmaceutical companies must often strike a balance between proper testing and pushing the drug to market. Unfortunately if the gamble fails, it can lead to loss or damage to human life.

Ethical Issue of Pharmaceutics During Drug Promotion

Drug promotion is an important part of pharmaceutical companies. They spend hundreds of millions of dollars on advertising to the public and to doctors. How can they sell their product if no one knows about it? Sounds like good business practice. However, when human health and human lives are at stake, normal business practices do no always apply, at least not without raising some major ethical concerns. While drug promotion to the public has some concerns, drug promotion to the doctors is a real concern. Through free lunches, free merchandise, and relatively high-pressured sale tactics, doctors are often bombarded with pharmaceutical drug representatives, who are attempting to convince the doctor to prescribe their new treatment. The problem arises due to these high-pressure sales: commercial businesses that are trying to gain a profit, are manipulating and to some degree are controlling healthcare, potentially altering how a doctor treats a patient.

Ethics Surrounding End-of-Life Care

In healthcare it is generally thought that patients' lives exceed all else, and many times doctors will go against the direct wishes of patients to save their lives. A patient will often need to have a "do not resuscitate" order, a legal blockade that doctors must follow, which ceases any life-saving techniques if vital signs fall below a certain point. The ethical question that involves much of end-of-life care surrounds the concept of quality of life versus quantity of life. Should a life be saved at all costs (a person with no readable brainwave activity be stuck in a bed for the rest of their life) or should quality of life be of importance as well? In general it is thought that healthcare personnel, pharmacists included, should do no harm. But the question that every person should ask themselves is this—"What does it mean to do harm to someone?"

Ethical Issues Surrounding the Individual Versus Society

One particular ethical dilemma that pharmacists and other healthcare personnel will have to face is the question of the **individual versus society**. This type of ethical dilemma can be observed when quarantining a patient with a very infectious disease. The patient's freedom is taken from them, sometimes against their wishes; however, this quarantine will save the life of many other people in society. One another example of this ethical dilemma can be observed in clinical trials, where some patients may be receiving less than ideal treatment, such as a placebo, rather than a new experimental drug. At one point this does not seem fair, that a patient would not be given a treatment that could potentially save their life, on the other hand, the experimental drug could one day be marketed and used to treat many sick patients if the experiment is performed properly and shows a strong safety and efficacy profile.

Randomized Drug Tests

Randomized drug tests are a rather effective means to control drug use and abuse. Many employers have adopted this type of test to deter drug abuse among their employees. Government agencies also use this form of drug testing, such as for police and firefighters. Randomized drug tests are also used in prisons, schools, and the military. This form of drug testing is used in healthcare and various businesses. There is significant success with this form of drug testing, however, there are many **controversies** surrounding this form of drug testing. Randomized drug testing is arguably unconstitutional and is thought to violate the fourth amendment which states that privacy of the person is protected from unwarranted search and seizure. To get past this, most companies will require agreement to randomized drug testing in some form, usually in a signed agreement before the employee is hired.

Oath of the Pharmacist

The **Oath of the Pharmacist of the American Pharmacists Association** is the promise given by the pharmacist on admission into the profession and outlines the vow the pharmacist makes in reference to service to others and the methods used to carry out the vow:

- Maintaining humanity's welfare and relief of suffering as primary concerns.
- Applying skills, knowledge and experience in order to produce optimal patient outcomes.
- Maintaining confidentiality in personal and health information.
- Accepting the responsibility of remaining current in knowledge and expertise.

- Maintaining high moral, ethical, and legal standards for the self and colleagues.
- Embracing changes that promote better patient care and outcomes.
- Mentoring the next generation of pharmacists.

Code of Ethics for Pharmacists

The Code of Ethics for Pharmacists of the American Pharmacists Associations contains a preamble (which identifies pharmacists and explains that the purpose of the code is to form the basis for the pharmacist's roles) and eight provisions and responsibilities required of the pharmacist:

1. Respecting the covenant between the patient and pharmacist: The pharmacist has a moral obligation to honor the trust of those receiving medication services.
2. Promoting patient good: The pharmacist always considers the needs of the patients.
3. Respecting patient autonomy: The pharmacist respects the patients' rights to self-determination and encourages them to participate in decision making.
4. Acting with honesty and integrity: The pharmacist is honest and acts without discrimination.
5. Maintaining professional competence: The pharmacist maintains education and remains current in the field of pharmacology.
6. Respecting values/abilities of colleagues and healthcare professionals: The pharmacist utilizes consultation and referral in the best interests of the patient.
7. Serving individual, community, and societal needs: The pharmacist recognizes obligations.
8. Seeking justice: The pharmacist exercises fairness in allocating health resources.

IRBs

The **Institutional Review Board** (IRB) is an independent ethics committee that has been designated to oversee human testing (clinical trials) at hospitals and research facilities. The IRB is empowered with important regulations by the United States department of Food and Drug Association (FDA) and the United States Department of Health and Human Services, allowing the IRB to approve or disapprove research as well as monitoring the validity and safety of the research. The safety of the patient is the IRB's most important focus. The research act of 1974 defines the regulatory powers of the IRB.

Belmont Report

The Belmont report was created by the United States department of Health and Human Services in 1979 and was an important document that provided guidelines for modern medical ethics. The Belmont report puts forth three important ethical components of human research that should be followed in any experiment. These include respect for the patients, always to strive to do well, and that all patients with similar disease states in the test should be treated the same without any bias.

Nuremberg Code

The Nuremberg code came about after the atrocities of the Nazis during World War II and came about during the Nuremberg trials. These codes were written in August of 1947 and are one of the first historical guidelines set out for human experiments and informed consent. These guidelines stated that people's consent must be obtained before a test is performed, tests must be socially valuable, intentional injury is not permitted (tests must be used to heal not hurt), animal studies must be performed first, all the research must be closely supervised, the benefits of the tests must always outweigh the risks, and tests must be ended as soon as it appears the experiments are causing more pain than help.

Factors to Address When Applying Evidence-Based Medicine to Actual Patients

When **applying evidenced-based medicine (EBM) in healthcare**, one should closely compare the patient with the subjects in the study. This is necessary to determine if the study is actually a valid option for treatment. If differing variables exist between the patients studied, such as different population subtype, different disease state, etc. this may lead to some issues when applying the EBM. It is also important to determine the cost-benefit ratio of the EBM when applied to the patient. Are possible risks and costs worth the possible benefit of the EBM that is suggested by the study? Finally, patients should be spoken to about the EBM in order to determine if the type of healthcare intervention that would be provided is something they feel comfortable with or agree to.

Ethical Justification for Use of Placebos

There are certain ethical considerations that should be met in a **clinical trial** before placebos should be used (although this does not mean that these considerations are always met before placebos are used in research). A placebo can be used: if there is no truly effective standard of treatment, the therapy is no better than a placebo, if recent evidence has suggested that the standard of treatment might be less than ideal and possibly dangerous, or if cost-effectiveness of using the treatment is not feasible for the entire patient population. It would always be best to compare new drugs to standard treatments. This will provide a better understanding of the treatments effectiveness and safety than against a placebo.

Health Care Systems

Health Care Financing in the US

Health care financing in the United States includes:

- **Private pay-for-service**: Those with no insurance coverage pay directly for services.
- **Private insurance**: The insurance company, paid for privately or through employment, pays an agreed upon amount or percentage of costs, and the insured may pay an agreed amount, such as a deductible for each visit or treatment.
- **Medicare**: Those who are over 65 or disabled and qualified are covered through this government program for 80% of customary and reasonable costs. Most Medicare insured also carry a private supplementary insurance to cover the remaining 20%.
- **Medicaid**: This combined federal and state welfare program authorized by Title XIX of the Social Security Act and regulated by the Centers for Medicare and Medicaid Services (CMS) assists people with low income with payment for medical care. This program provides assistance for all ages, including children.
- **Veteran's health care benefits**: Provides health care for veteran's and some dependents based on priorities, with those having ≥50% service-related disabilities priority one.
- **Tricare**: Provides coverage for health care to service members and their dependents.

US Health Care System vs. That of Other Nations

Healthcare models in other nations:

Model	Nations	Description
Beveridge	Great Britain, New Zealand, Spain, Cuba, Scandinavian countries	Government is sole payer and owns most medical facilities. Physicians may be public or private.

Model	Nations	Description
Bismarck	Germany, Belgium, France, Japan, Switzerland, Netherlands	People have insurance through employers and pay part of cost. Everyone must enroll.
National Health Insurance	Canada, South Korea, Taiwan	Single payer system into which everyone must contribute. Government is sole payer but healthcare providers are private.
Out-of-Pocket	Most of the developing world (India, Cambodia)	Pay as you go with money or goods or go without care.
Mixed model	United States	VA health is similar to Beveridge model; Medicare to National Health, employer-provided insurance to Bismarck. Uninsured, like out-of-pocket.

Medicare

Medicare is a federally run health insurance agency entitled to all men and women that are American citizens or permanent residents over the age of 65. Medicare is also available for some people with disabilities that are younger than 65 such as people with renal failure. There are four categories of benefits offered by Medicare: parts A, B, C, and D. Part A benefits cover hospital stays and in certain cases nursing home stays. Plan B covers outpatient therapies, X-rays therapies, doctor visits, dialysis, chemotherapy, wheelchairs, prosthetic devices, etc. Part C allows beneficiaries to get coverage under private health plans. Part D addresses prescription drug costs. Medicare only provides some payment for any of its benefits and out-of-pocket payment is also required for services, which can include deductibles and co-payments.

Medicaid

Medicaid is a low-income joint federal-state health insurance plan. Federal government and state governments pay for this program. The federal government offers grants; more money goes to states in more need, less to richer states. Although the federal government regulates the main underlying rules of Medicaid, each state differs a little in eligibility and how the program is handled. Medicaid allows for low-income citizens and permanent residents, although other requirements may be necessary depending on state laws, to receive health benefits. Medicaid covers generally more benefits the other US healthcare system, Medicare. Medicaid, however, does not consistently cover psychologists, physical therapy or podiatrists (this coverage varies by state).

HMOs

HMO is known as **Health Maintenance Organization** and it is a type of Managed Care in which health insurance is provided through a private organization. HMOs work generally through contracts with specific doctors and hospitals. By providing some doctors more patients, an HMO can receive discounts on medical care, leading to cheaper costs for the patients of this insurance. There are generally three types of HMOs: staff model HMO, group model, and network model. In the staff model, doctors are under employment of the HMO. They work in buildings owned by the HMO and may only see patients that belong to an HMO insurance Plan. In the group model, the HMO pays and contracts with an established group of doctors, not individual doctors, to provide care for HMO patients for fee for service. In the independent practice association model, HMOs make contracts with individual doctors and practices, in which the doctor will see HMO members, but will also see other non-HMO patients as well. In the Network Model, HMO contracts with groups, individual practices, etc. to create a large network of doctors that will care for HMO patients.

Medically Indigent Patient

Identifying the **medically indigent patient** in the United States is a difficult task. This is due in part to the fact that many people who are medically indigent are often homeless, do not speak English or are not legal residents of the USA. Additionally, the definition of medically indigent is relative and up for debate, but is usually defined as a patient that does not have any type of health insurance. This definition is somewhat flawed as it will exclude patients that have minimal health insurance. Typically, the medically indigent population is estimated using surveys from healthcare organizations and hospitals. Criteria that are used in these surveys include annual patient income, the age of the patient, and the race of the patient.

Healthcare Issues

While it is known that the United States does not have universal healthcare, it is often assumed that the poor healthcare indigent population is medically covered via Medicaid. Unfortunately, this is often not the case due to budgeting issues and the fact that every state can define eligibility to their Medicaid programs. Additionally, it is often difficult to specifically assess how many people in any specific state are potentially in need of state medical support. This is due to the fact that while much of the population has no or inadequate insurance, they do not request state support until a major health related crisis occurs.

Role of Pharmacology in Chronic Disease Prevention and Health Promotion

Pharmacology has an important role in **chronic disease prevention and health promotion**. Because pharmacists work in many settings and have access to many patients, pharmacists can take an active role in primary prevention efforts through efforts at educating the public about disease. Patients are often unaware of the importance of immunizations in preventing disease, especially in adulthood when, for example, the herpes zoster vaccines may prevent the disease altogether or lessen its severity. The pharmacist should point out to patients the importance of annual influenza vaccinations. The pharmacist may offer screenings, such as blood pressure, as part of secondary prevention. Additionally, pharmacists have an active role in tertiary prevention: Many people do not understand the importance of adhering to medication protocols for the treatment of one disorder in order to prevent development of a more serious disorder, such as treating hypertension to prevent heart failure or stroke. Patients may take medications haphazardly or omit or reduce dosages, not understanding that these changes may have implications.

Decreasing the Levels of Microbial Outbreaks and Microbial Resistance in Hospitals

Arguably one of the most important steps to remember and to teach fellow hospital colleagues is proper **sterile technique**:

1. Washing the hands thoroughly.
2. Quarantine patients that have microbial infections in order to decrease possible spread of disease, particularly if the microbial infection is resistant.
3. Do not prescribe antimicrobial drugs unless absolutely necessary. Improper prescription of these drugs can quickly lead to the generation of resistant microbial strains.
4. Use broad-spectrum antibiotics as an initial defense, but adjust therapy appropriately and use narrower spectrum antibiotics as more becomes known about the underlying infection.
5. Educate health care colleagues, doctors and staff on microbials and antimicrobials, including the proper selection of antimicrobial drugs during diagnosis of the infection.
6. Understand the patterns of resistance of antimicrobials in your hospital. Combining these steps can help prevent spread and increased resistance of microbials as well as leading to promoting more effective diagnosis and therapy.

Pharmacoeconomics

Balance Sheet Accounts

There are three accounts used to measure changes between a pharmacy's worth and its debt. These types of accounts are known as **balance sheet accounts** and they include assets, liabilities and equity. Assets are the commodities that the individual, or in this case the pharmacy, owns. Assets can include the drugs on the shelves, as well as the company itself. Assets can generally be sold or changed into cash. Liabilities are what an individual owes; this can include rent, investments, credit toward a specific service, etc. Liabilities at some time must be paid back. Convertible value means that theoretically you could sell the item for cash, such as a house or stocks. Equity is also known as net worth. This tells a company if they actually are in the red (debt) or in the black (made profit). Equity is what is left over after all liabilities are subtracted from the assets. Any company, pharmacy or otherwise, should have a greater number of assets than liabilities, thus greater equity.

Intangible Costs

These are costs that do not have a measurable financial or economic basis, but are instead costs that are felt in direct response to a disease. **Intangible costs** are not quantitative measurements, but instead they are qualitative. However, they are as important in measuring as more quantitative economic measurements. Intangible costs include pain, guilt, general suffering, and grief due to a certain disease. These costs should always be taken into account when making healthcare decisions.

Direct Medical Costs and Direct Nonmedical Costs

Direct medical costs are costs of medical therapies including drugs, hospital stays, diagnostic tests, salaries for physicians and pharmacists, and other healthcare costs. Direct medical costs can be divided into fixed costs and variable costs. Fixed costs include necessities such as rent and utilities. Generally, fixed costs do not rely on fluctuations that are observed with changes in medical treatments: these costs remain stable. Variable costs change in response to need. For example, the greater amount a diagnostic test or treatment is performed, the greater amount of the cost. If certain drugs are needed at a higher level, for example, in a particular month, then the variable cost for the drug during that month would be greater. **Direct nonmedical costs** can include costs that are in response to an illness but not necessarily medically related, such as gas for the trip to the hospital, ambulance ride, special diets, etc.

Income and Expense Accounts

Income accounts involve the payment or other assets received for the services provided to the customer. The income accounts can be individual, in the sense of a paycheck. Income accounts can also relate to the actual assets earned by a company, money gained, for example, for selling a certain product. **Expense accounts involve** money that is used to buy things. In a pharmacy this relate to buying pharmaceuticals, paying employees etc. For the individual this can relate to buying a car, food, or paying for rent. If income is higher than expenses, then the company or individual made a profit. If the expenses are higher than income, then they are in debt.

Indirect Non-Medical Costs

Indirect non-medical costs are costs in response to illness, such as loss of workdays and loss of salary. There are generally two means to measure indirect costs, which include human capital (HC) and willingness to pay techniques (WTP). The HC technique attempts to measure the value of a person's life in relation to their level of income. The WTP technique uses a method by which the patient is asked how much they would be willing to pay to treat a disease. The WTP technique asks the patients how much their health and life are worth, while the HC technique just assumes how valuable it is. These measurements are very important, however, very subjective.

Opportunity Costs

Opportunity costs occur when a certain alternative treatment no longer becomes an option for treatment due to another treatment choice that may have been made. An example of an opportunity cost occurs when someone belongs to a certain health insurance company or HMO, which usually have specific medical formularies for specific medical treatments or drug prescriptions that must be followed in order to receive the healthcare benefit. Often due to monetary reasons, most people must stick with their health insurance company's formulary, losing opportunities to take other drugs or medical treatments, even if the alternative treatment is more beneficial and effective for treating the disease.

Prospective Reimbursement and Retrospective Reimbursement

Prospective reimbursement is when someone pays in advance for a service. This is similar to when someone, for example, buys a plane ticket before they fly on the plane, or when someone pays a healthcare premiums or a monthly health insurance fee before they can receive benefits from the health insurance. **Retrospective reimbursement** occurs when someone pays after a service has been rendered. This can be seen with a lot of the economy. When someone goes to a restaurant, most of the time they pay after they get their food. In a pharmacy, a patient will pay for their prescription after it has been filled and properly counted for them.

Cost-Minimization Analysis

Cost-minimization analysis is a pharmacoeconomic tool that analyzes the net cost of two different medical treatments, assuming that everything else (safety, efficacy, etc.) is equal. An example of this is performed when attempting to analyze the net cost of two different drugs, a name brand and generic brand for example, which show equal effectiveness of treating a certain disease state as well as equal safety comparing two different drugs that are bioequivalent, showing equal efficacy and safety. This analysis can help minimize costs with equivalent therapy.

Cost-Effective Analysis

Cost-effective analysis **(CEA)** is a pharmacoeconomic technique to compare two or more medical treatments for relative efficacy, safety, as well as cost. Generally, in a pharmacy, a ratio comparing changes in cost versus changes in efficacy of two or more different drugs is used. This ratio is known as the incremental cost-effectiveness ratio (ICER).

$$\mathbf{ICER} = \frac{\mathbf{Cost\ of\ drug\ A - Cost\ of\ drug\ B}}{\mathbf{Efficacy\ of\ drug\ A - Efficacy\ of\ drug\ B}}$$

Perspectives of Pharmacoeconomics

Societal

The **societal perspective** of pharmacoeconomics is a very extensive subject and generally consists of all other perspectives: patient, payer and provider. This perspective uses a broader outlook of general consequences of medicine and is important in places and countries that have governmentally controlled healthcare. Other important costs include patient death rate, as well as general costs needed for healthcare. Some view this perspective as the important perspective when studying pharmacoeconomics.

PATIENT

The **patient perspective** of pharmacoeconomics considers the following questions:

- How does the patient view the cost of the drug or medical treatment?
- How much will the patient pay?
- What effect will this have on the patient's quality of life?

These questions are necessary when attempting to understand the pharmacoeconomics of healthcare. Patients are the basis for all healthcare and it is important to understand the cost that a patient will pay and what effect this will have on their views of healthcare. High payment in the eyes of patient is often a huge reason to not pursue proper healthcare.

PROVIDER

Providers of healthcare include hospitals, HMO organizations and private practices that diagnose and treat various diseases of patients. These organizations have a lot of payments and costs to maintain the functionality of the healthcare field. Direct cost of drugs, managed care, short-term and long-term hospital care, diagnostic tests and salaries are a few examples of costs that the providers of healthcare must pay and are an important pharmacoeconomic consideration when determining the overall cost of a particular medical treatment.

PAYER

Those that are considered **payers** are employers, government, and insurance companies, which often include insurance companies that are reimbursed by the employer of the patient. These types of costs are often direct in the sense that the company, employer or government, pays for the patients healthcare. Other indirect costs to the payer can include loss of work from the sick employee, loss of revenue due to loss of productivity. This perspective is often considered when a company or employer contracts with a specific health care plan such as an HMO.

HUMANISTIC OUTCOMES IN RELATION TO PHARMACEUTICALS

Humanistic outcomes (i.e., health-related quality-of-life outcomes) refer to those outcomes that result from disease or treatment (such as drug therapy) on the patient's functional status or overall quality of life. The focus remains on the patient's perspective rather than on reports of mortality and morbidity. Functional status considerations include:

- **Physical**: Mobility, energy level, pain, performance level.
- **Psychological**: Anxiety, depression, cognitive functioning, behavior, control.
- **Social**: Relationships, participation, community resources, standard of living, employment, levels of satisfaction.

Humanistic outcomes also focus on perceptions of health, such as belief systems about the causes of disease. Humanistic outcomes are most often assessed with tools, such as questionnaires, which may be general or disease-specific, such as an instrument for patients with diabetes mellitus, type I. Instruments with visual analog scales are easy for patients to complete and can generally be done quickly, increasing participation rates. The pharmacist may ask patients to complete a self-administered written test during contact. Personal interviews may be influenced by bias and response is often poor to mailed questionnaires.

Population-Based Care, Pharmacoepidemiology, and Public Health

Importance of Pharmacoepidemiology in Writing Prescriptions and Counseling Patients

Pharmacoepidemiology is generally used to study adverse reactions of drugs in the population. Pharmacoepidemiology is not used to lessen adverse reactions, necessarily. Although pharmacoepidemiology can be used to remove potentially dangerous drugs from the market, adverse reactions will always happen. A bigger reason for post-market surveillance is to study the rate of adverse reactions so that physicians can be more informed and write better, smarter and safer prescriptions. Additionally, pharmacoepidemiology can be used to provide more counseling points for pharmacists to provide patients, increasing the possible safety of the therapy for the patients.

Pharmacovigilance

Pharmacovigilance is a subarea of pharmacoepidemiology, which monitors and reports on adverse effects and other safety related aspects of drugs that are already on the market. This type of measurement is used in phase IV clinical trials. Often reports of adverse effects are given by healthcare personnel. The FDA has websites for reporting adverse effects of drugs that may have been missed in pre-market clinical trials. Also since many drugs have shown adverse toxicities during post-market clinical trials, such as Vioxx, the FDA is making tighter regulations about post-market studies on the safety of the drugs and adverse reactions.

FAERS

The US Food and Drug Administration (FDA) maintains the **FDA Adverse Event Reporting System** (FAERS) database as part of the safety surveillance of drugs after they are marketed as well as other products: prescription and OTC medications, biologics, medical devices, combination productions, nutritional products (infant formula, medical foods), cosmetics, and food/beverages. The database contains reports of (1) adverse events, (2) medication errors, (3) product quality complaints associated with adverse events. Reports are evaluated to determine if further study is indicated. Reports may be submitted by any healthcare professional (including pharmacists), consumers (patients, families, others), and manufacturers. Reports are submitted through the MedWatch website, which provides forms that can be downloaded as well as online reporting forms. Medwatch provides links to the Safety Reporting Panel to file concerns about tobacco and to the Vaccine Adverse Event Reporting Systems (VAERS) to report concerns about vaccines as these are not reported to FAERS.

NCC MERP

The independent **National Coordinating Counsel for Medication Error Reporting and Prevention (NCC MERP)** comprises 27 different national organizations that have collaborated in order to identify the causes of medication errors and to promote safety in medication use through voluntary reporting. NCC MERP provides a standard definition of medication errors, a standard taxonomy of medication errors to use in the development of databases, and a medication error index, which classifies medications errors into 9 categories:

1. Circumstances/Events that may lead to error.
2. Error occurred but did not directly affect patient.
3. Error occurred and reached patient but caused no harm.
4. Error occurred, reached patient, and required some intervention to prevent harm.
5. Error occurred that may have or did cause temporary harm and required some intervention.

6. Error occurred that may have or did cause temporary harm and required initial or prolonged hospitalization.
7. Error occurred that may have or did cause permanent patient harm.
8. Error occurred that required prolonged intervention to sustain life.
9. Error may have or did result in patient's death.

Limitations of Pre-Marketing Clinical Trials

There are many **limitations of pre-marketing clinical trials**, also known as phase I, phase II, and phase III clinical trials, which make it necessary to perform post-marketing pharmacoepidemiological studies, an important component of the pharmaceutical industry. These limitations include short duration of the clinical trials, small population subset (these clinical trials often do not test on a group representative of total population that might benefit from this drugs use), and small sample size (only tests a small group of people, a lot of important data about the drug's safety can go unnoticed by the researchers and drug manufacturers). Additionally, new drugs are often compared only to placebos and not presently available drugs to determine if this drug truly is safer and has more efficacy than the already marketed drugs. Post-market studies can be helpful in studying the safety of the drugs as well as the cost-benefit ratio of the drug compared to other marketed therapies.

QALYs

QALY stands for **Quality-Adjusted Life Years**, a measurement of quality years of life that medical intervention could provide a patient. The years added to a person's life are coded with number between 1 (healthy) and 0 (dead). If medical intervention provides a patient with extra healthy years, then it is considered to be worth the risk or the cost to intervene. However, if the patient's extra years are less than ideal, for example if they would live in pain, then each year of their life would be given a number generally less than one, which gives an indication of quality of life in relationship to length of life. The variables that are used to determine the quality of life include time-trade off (what a patient prefers, a long sick life, or short healthy life), gamble (if the patient had a choice would they choose to gamble on a medical therapy (drug regimen) that may potentially cure them or kill them, visual analog scale (having patients rate a certain illness between 100 and 0, 0 = death, 100 = perfect health).

Studies in Pharmacoepidemiology

Cohort Studies

Cohort studies are commonly used in pharmacoepidemiology. A cohort study is a longitudinal correlation study. In medicine it is generally used to find correlative data between causes and disease states as well as correlative data between drugs and adverse reactions. A cohort study generally compares two groups of people, for example one group who has been receiving a particular treatment, while the other group would not be receiving any treatment. These studies were not as accurate as randomized control studies used in clinical trials, because the groups in a cohort study are not always controlled properly, and many variables might exist between the populations. However, in such cases of studying adverse reactions in connection to a certain drug therapy, it is not considered ethical to measure by randomized control studies. Cohort studies can be very long, and with that other challenges exist, like unforeseen changes within the groups including death and development of new diseases. Cohort studies are thought to be better than case-controlled studies.

Case-Controlled Studies

Case-controlled studies are a method used in pharmacoepidemiology. Case-control studies are less expensive than other studies and usually smaller and more manageable by smaller lab groups.

Case-controlled studies are considered retrospective, in that "cases", such as medical files for patients who have a specific disease state or specific drug therapy, are compared back to control groups (patients who do not have the disease or not on the drug therapy). These studies are good relatively cheap and fast studies to measure toxicity of drugs and various other adverse reactions. Although they are more accurate than some studies (cross-sectional studies), they are not as accurate as cohort studies.

Cross-Sectional Studies

Cross-sectional studies are a way to study all points or members of a population at a given point in time. This type of study is one of the least accurate of pharmacoepidemiological studies, however, provides a reasonable idea of relationships among the population at a given-time point. Surveys, for example, are often a good example of a cross-sectional study. Another example of a cross-sectional study would be a hypothesis that drug x caused renal failure. If the researchers in this study found that a significantly greater amount of people at a given point in time had renal failure that were taking drug X, the hypothesis would be supported. However, cross-sectional studies do not look at variables as they change in time. They generally miss a lot more data that other pharmacoepidemiological studies.

Continuous Quality Improvement

Quality Assurance in Drug Compounding

Quality assurance develops measurements, standards, practices, and critical indicators for the use of drugs in compounding, storage, dispensing, and other aspects of medication preparation and use in a pharmacy. Using quality assurance documents in each process helps to identify emerging areas of improvement or need, and provides solutions to problems. Documentation practices include correctly capturing data (written and electronic) for the receipt, storage, use, and disposal of each drug. Another type of documentation is labeling. Each solution, compounded mixture, or any other container that contains an active or inert ingredient must be label with the name of the ingredient, date of preparation, expiration date, concentration, and initials of the operator.

Bar-Code and Data Entry Technologies

Each product has a unique scannable bar code that is linked to its National Drug Code (NDC) number. During the dispensing process, the bar code of each stock bottle is scanned to ensure that it matches the NDC number dispensed. Drug bar codes are also scanned when they are loaded into automated dispensing robots or cabinets (e.g., Pyxis machines). This helps ensure that the correct medication is loaded into the correct container, drawer, or pocket. When medications are loaded into or dispensed from an automated dispensing system, inventory levels are also updated. This helps ensure that the correct on-hand inventory for each medication is maintained in the computer system.

Data entry technologies are also used by pharmacies for quality assurance. Many pharmacy computer systems allow new prescriptions to be scanned into the system, and most of the prescription details are prefilled. In most hospitals, prescribers order medications using the same software that the pharmacy uses to dispense medications. Therefore, medication aides can pull prescription details from the computer system without manually entering the information. This reduces the risk of human error. Additionally, the computer system will usually automatically select preferred formulary products that are in stock at the pharmacy.

Pyrogen Testing

A pyrogen is any substance that causes an inflammatory response and manifests in an increase in body temperature. Quality testing of pharmaceutical products involves pyrogen testing to ensure patient safety. A form of pyrogen, endotoxin, is produced by bacteria and is known as the limulus amebocyte lysate (LAL) test. Another test to measure pyrogen, the rabbit test, is an *in vivo* test. Another test for pyrogens is the bacterial endotoxins test (BET), which is the most sensitive test. It is important to note that bacteria do not have to be alive to illicit an immune response in a patient—they only have to be present in the pharmaceutical drug product in high enough numbers to cause a reaction. Endotoxin is a very small substance that will pass through a 0.2 micron filter, which autoclaving will not depyrogenate.

Social Determinants of Health

Social determinants of health refer to the non-medical elements of a person's social environment that have a direct impact on his or her physical health and tendencies. The heavy influence of this component of health is reflected in its being listed as one of the five main sections of *Healthy People 2030.* According to HHS, social determinants of health are "the conditions in the environments where people are born, live, learn, work, play, worship, and age that affect a wide range of health, functioning, and quality-of-life outcomes and risks." For these reasons, a health history should inquire into the patient's social determinants of health also:

- The patient's **lifestyle** is an important component of the patient's health history and includes habits, diet, sleep, hobbies, and the patient's ability to perform the activities of daily living.
- A **social history** is the component of the patient's health history that details family relationships, ethnicity, educational level, economic status, and the condition of the patient's home and environment.
- The patient's health history also includes the patient's **psychological status** and the patient's **usual means of obtaining healthcare.**

Pharmacy Practice Management

Pharmacy Benefit Manager

A pharmacy benefit manager is a company that is under contract with HMOs, government programs, and other insured healthcare companies to regulate numerous important things including developing and regulating of a prescription drug formulary for insurance companies. They are also useful in contracting various pharmacies and obtaining drug discounts for the insurance companies from drug manufacturers. These companies are responsible for drug utilization reviews and they can also help set-up mail order pharmacies for the insurance companies.

DEA 222 Order Form

Orders of scheduled or controlled drugs, classes I and II, require the use of a **DEA 222 order** form. Each drug order requires three copies of the DEA 222 order form. Each DEA 222 order has ten lines, one line per drug. On each line is the drug name, dosage form and number of drugs or volume of the drug in each container. The form must be filled out completely and accurately, or it will be sent back without being ordered. Two of the three copies go to the supplier of the drug; the third copy is kept by the pharmacy. The supplier holds onto one copy of the DEA form 222 and the last form is sent to the DEA. Upon receiving the order, the pharmacy must record all the drugs on the form that they received and keep it for the pharmacy records.

DEA 41 Form

Damaged, expired, and unwanted class II controlled drugs must be accounted for and disposed of properly. In order to dispose of a drug, the **DEA 41 form** must be filled out in triplicate, with two copies sent to the DEA and one kept in the pharmacy's records for the minimum of two years after disposal of the drug. The records must include the DEA number, name and address of the pharmacist/pharmacy, the reverse distributors DEA number, name and address, and the amount of drug and means of disposal. **Disposal of the drug** is generally handled in three ways.:

1. Contact the original supplier of the drug: some will take back the drug. This is the easiest way for disposal.
2. Onsite disposal if disposed drugs are less than one pound is overseen by a representative from the DEA.
3. For quantities greater than one pound, a reverse distributor must be used. A reverse distributor is generally a DEA approved company that will resell or properly dispose of drug compounds.

DEA 106 Form

When dealing with a controlled substance it is vital for the pharmacy to keep exact records for their controlled drugs and to be able to account for all drugs in their inventory and all drugs that have been prescribed. All controlled drugs must be kept secure according to the DEA. All CII drugs must be kept secure, usually in a locked cabinet that is firmly secured to a wall. If a drug is lost or stolen, even if only one pill, **a DEA form 106** must be filled out. The form must be submitted to the DEA within 10 days. Failure to report any lost or theft of a drug can lead to steep penalties and fines.

Drug Utilization Reviews

Drug utilization reviews are performed by hospitals and retail pharmacies, in which data is collected on drug utilization or drug use patterns. These reviews, when performed in a hospital, can give ideas of how much drugs are used, if the drugs are being used properly according to hospital protocols, and of the safety and efficacy of a given therapy. Commercial pharmacies often use drug utilization reviews to study which drugs are most popular or "fast-moving" and to try to keep these drugs stocked in the pharmacy. Additionally, these reviews can be used to determine the expense being paid for a certain popular drug, if it is very expensive for the pharmacy as well as the patient, the pharmacy can use this data to push toward prescribing an equally effective and safe generic version of the same drug.

Importance of Location of Pharmacy

A **major principle of marketing is location**: the place of business must be positioned in an area that has heavy traffic for people that would be interested in your product. It has occurred countless times, a business that has a great product and good prices has gone bankrupt because the location was not feasible for their clientele to reach. For example, if you have a pharmacy in a region that caters to a more geriatric (elderly) clientele, having the pharmacy on the top of a steep hill might not be the best option, as they would find it difficult to reach the pharmacy.

Advantages and Disadvantages of Promoting a Pharmacy in Different Venues

Promotion of the pharmacy is a way to advertise about prices and services provided. Advertisements include television, radio, newspaper and internet ads. All forms of advertising have their advantages and disadvantages. In radio and television, ads can reach a greater number of people, but are usually more expensive and must have a relatively mass appeal for the cost of the advertisements to match the possible benefit. Newspapers are generally cheaper and they can generally reach a pretty large audience, however, the audience is smaller than that of television or radio. With the internet, a relatively massive amount of people can be reached at a very small cost in the guise of pop-up ads, website sponsors, and email; however, many people view this type of advertising as a nuisance. Additionally, word of mouth, happy customers telling other people of your business, is often one of the most effective, cheapest (free), yet limited forms of advertisement. All it takes is a good product and a good customer service.

Important Objectives to Meet When Setting Prices

Properly **pricing products** and **services** is an important aspect of pharmacy marketing. If too expensive, customers will not purchase anything. If the prices are too cheap, the pharmacy will not make enough money to remain in business. It is important to set up a pricing regimen that will maintain a stable income while maintaining competitive prices. Pricing is also considered based on the original cost of the product as well as demand of the product. While it is wise to have prices lower than or equal to competition, the price shouldn't be lower than the original cost of the product, otherwise the pharmacy would never thrive. Additionally if a certain product becomes very popular or there is a high demand for it, this can be a reason to increase the price, which will both take care of the higher cost of having a greater supply of the product as well as increasing profit potential, as long as the price is not terribly different from the competition.

Pharmacist's Roles

Hospital Setting

A **pharmacist's role in the hospital setting** can be extremely varied. In the hospital setting, a pharmacist generally has two major roles: core pharmacist and clinical pharmacist. When a pharmacist is working in the core pharmacy, they are responsible for inputting and checking orders, answering physician questions, monitoring parenteral products being mixed by technicians and if needed, helping to respond to emergency codes. When a pharmacist is a clinical pharmacist, they are typically working in close contact with the medical staff. Often, the clinical pharmacist goes on rounds with the medical team and directly monitors medication profiles for each patient. Clinical pharmacist will also provide antibiotic and anticoagulation monitoring. Many doctors in a hospital setting will have pharmacists provide all vancomycin and aminoglycoside dosing and monitoring. Most pharmacists who work in a hospital rotate through various shifts and will switch between working in the core pharmacy and working on the floor.

Retail or Community Pharmacy Setting

In a **retail or community pharmacy setting**, the pharmacist has several very important roles. It is very important to remember that a pharmacist in a community setting is often the last medical professional that a patient may see. This means that it is vital that a pharmacist working in the community makes sure that all medicine related questions are thoroughly answered. This includes new medication counseling and taking the time to make sure the patient does not have any questions related to medications the patient is already taking. Additional duties of a community pharmacist include: prescription checking, answering medicine related questions from physicians and patients, providing vaccination services, monitoring medication interactions, and providing any additional medication counseling and training as needed. Retail and community pharmacies can range from very small community pharmacies that have a very specific longstanding patient base and fill as little as 50 prescriptions a day to very large chain store retail pharmacies that fill over a thousand prescriptions a day.

Role of Pharmacy Manager in Personnel Management

The role of the pharmacy manager in **personnel management** includes:

- **Hiring and firing**: Ensuring individuals are qualified and do not have a history of drug abuse and verifying history of employment. Exercising fairness in hiring and avoiding discrimination. Taking steps to fire individuals for legitimate cause when necessary.
- **Scheduling**: Ensuring that all staff members have equitable schedules and accounting for sick time, vacation time, holidays, and personal time off.
- **Training**: Providing training on site specific activities within the person's appropriate scope of practice.
- **Supervising**: Ensuring that staff members are carrying out duties appropriately and have the education, training, and tools they need to function effectively. Conducting annual performance reviews.
- **Handling conflicts**: Preventing exacerbation of disagreements.
- **Mentoring**: Providing guidance to others in the field of pharmacy.
- **Promoting teamwork**: Outlining the need for teams and providing a model for teamwork.

Business Planning and Strategic Planning

Business planning requires a focus on the needs of an organization currently and in the near future in regards to marketing and production. Business planning includes assessing budgetary constraints, determining products and services, conducting or reviewing a market survey, developing marketing strategies, and reviewing organizational needs as well as potential risk factors that may impact services/production. **Strategic planning** requires a focus on needs of the organization, community, and customers and establish goals for not only the near future (2–4 years) but into the extended future (10–15 years). Strategic planning must be based on assessments, both internal and external, to determine the present courses of action, needed changes, priorities, and methodologies to effect change. The focus of strategic planning must be on development of services based on identified customer needs and then the marketing of those services. Organization-wide strategic planning includes collecting data, analyzing services/functions, identifying key issues, and developing revised mission and vision statement, specific goals, and objectives.

Accounting and Financial Elements of Pharmacy Management

Pharmacy management includes:

- **Budget**: Setting up and managing different types of budgets (operating, capital, cash balance, and master) by establishing accountability, controlling expenses, monitoring costs, and developing corrective action plans for problem areas. Staff members must be paid and money budgeted for benefit packages. Orders must be generated based on cash balance and bills paid in a timely manner.
- **Inventory**: Determining how much inventory to keep on hand and what levels trigger purchase is an important consideration in controlling costs. Money invested to improve inventory accounting may save money in the long term.
- **Audits**: Accuracy in accounting procedures must be ensured for both business and legal reasons and the cash flow balance carefully monitored to prevent deficit spending.
- **Reporting**: Financial reporting must be accurate and carried out according to schedule. For example, income taxes must be calculated correctly and paid on schedule to avoid penalties. Accounting reports may need to be presented to the administration or board of directors.

Risk Management

Risk management is an organized and formal method of decreasing liability, financial loss, and risk or harm to patients, staff, or others by doing an assessment of risk and introducing risk management strategies. Much of risk management has been driven by the insurance industry in order to minimize costs, but quality management utilizes risk management as a method to ensure quality healthcare and process improvement. Pharmaceutical practices are central to risk management because of risks inherent in medical treatment. The organization's risk management program usually comprises a manager and staff with a number of responsibilities:

- **Risk identification** begins with an assessment of processes to identify and prioritize those that require further study to determine risk exposure.
- **Risk analysis** requires a careful documenting of process, utilizing flow charts, with each step in the process assessed for potential risks. This may utilize root cause analysis methods.
- **Risk prevention** involves instituting corrective or preventive processes. Responsible individual or teams are identified and trained.
- **Assessment/evaluation** of corrective/preventive processes is ongoing to determine if they are effective or require modification.

Professional Communication

Verbal Communication

Communication is vital for healthcare when purveying important information to patients as well as colleagues about potential diagnostic therapies and medication. **Verbal communication** consists of spoken words but also can consist of written words as well. It is essential when speaking to a patient, for example, during counseling of a new prescription, to make sure the patient understands what is being said, to speak clearly and answer a lot of open-ended questions to make sure the patient understands about the drugs. It is also essential for written instructions on a medicine to be clear and easily understandable. Confusing written instructions can easily be a serious problem with a patient needing to follow a specific prescription.

Empathetic Communication Between Pharmacist and Patient

Empathetic communication includes active listening (showing respect and focusing on what the other person is saying) and acknowledging the emotions that the patients/families are exhibiting or expressing ("I can see how upset you are") rather than ignoring them. The pharmacist often encounters patients and family members when they are at their most vulnerable, such as when they are hospitalized or have been diagnosed with a disease, which may be serious or life-threatening. Patients and families may be anxious and fearful, and this may translate at times into anger, impatience, or withdrawal, so the pharmacist must be tolerant and patient in interactions with patients/families. The pharmacist must avoid appearing rushed and allow the patients/families the time they need to ask questions and fully understand the information the pharmacist is providing. The pharmacist should take the time to point out and explain important information, such as the need to take a medication on an empty stomach, and should provide information about pharmacy assistance programs when needed.

Nonverbal Communication

Nonverbal communication is also very important in healthcare. Nonverbal communication consists of techniques that do not require spoken or written words to get a particular meaning across. Nonverbal communications consist of kinesics, a technique that uses body language to convey a message, whether intentional or unintentional. Body language can include changes in posture, nervous tics, etc. Unintentional nervous tics can nonverbally tell a doctor or pharmacist a lot about a patient's state of mind and can help a lot with further verbal communication, in treatment, and in understanding the patient.

SOAP Notes

SOAP notes are a form of documentation used by pharmacists, physicians, and various other healthcare personnel to write and communicate about a patient. SOAP (subjective, objective, assessment and plan) notes are used to organize diagnostic results, physician and pharmacist orders, and other important notes about a patient or certain medical problems of a patient.

- **Subjective data** are problems and symptoms of a disease as described by the patient.
- **Objective data** are observations of a disease, symptoms, lab tests, etc. that are made by healthcare personnel about a disease.
- **Assessment data** consists of the judgment about a disease based on the objective and subjective data by the healthcare personnel (physicians).
- The **plan** of the soap note is the therapy action chosen based on the assessment of the disease.

SOAP notes provide a quick and organized way to assess and treat a patient, which is vital when working in a hospital with many diverse patients.

Key Points in Patient Profiles That Must Be Documented by Pharmacists

Do not forget that, as a pharmacist, you are a vital part of the healthcare continuum and as such it is vital that you document patient information and patient encounters. Ideally, every encounter you have with a patient should be documented in the **patient's permanent file**. If you are working in a hospital or group setting where you have access to the patient's electronic medical record, you should document patient encounters in the pharmacy notes section of the medical record. When you are documenting patient encounters always provide: a brief history of present illness (HPI), relevant prescriptions, drug allergies, assessment, plan and any other piece of information that is relevant to that specific encounter.

Effective Communication Between Pharmacist and Medical Team During Hospital Rounds

Effective communication is vital when there is limited time to present pertinent information about a patient to the **medical team**. Rounds or morning rounds is usually the only time when each patient case is discussed with the entire medical team. It is important that the pharmacist has reviewed each patient that is going to be discussed during rounds for medication related problems. This includes reviewing pertinent lab values and performing any antibiotic kinetics before rounds. Questions that need to be directed to the medical team should be formulated before rounds if possible, especially if a primary literature search is necessary. During rounds, pharmacist questions should be asked succinctly to the medical team and primary literature should be presented if asked for. If someone on the medical teams asks you a question about a patient that you cannot answer appropriately, you should offer to look up the information after rounds are complete. It is better to give physicians a more complete answer slightly after rounds than an incomplete answer during rounds.

Concordance

Concordance is a term that was recently coined describing the evolution of healthcare, particularly the relationship between patients, physicians and pharmacists in relation to the patients prescribed treatments. Concordance, in many ways, is like an oral contract between a patient and their healthcare providers that they will adhere to prescribed therapy as directed. This approach to healthcare makes patients more responsible for their well-being and not solely a responsibility of the physicians and pharmacists.

Perception of Pharmacists by Fellow Healthcare Colleagues

Pharmacists are an important component of healthcare; however, trust must be earned. It is important to be respectful to the healthcare team, keep them informed of important lab values and drug information of the patient. Pharmacists should be readily available to look up important primary literature to answer any questions that a physician or other healthcare personnel might have on a given case. A pharmacist should be willing to stand firm about a treatment of a patient, physicians might be overlooking a key component necessary in the treatment of the patient. It is also wise to know when to pick your battles and that at times realize that compromise is necessary. Older doctors unfortunately often are not always amenable to pharmacist intervention, partially for the reason that the role of a pharmacist has evolved greatly in recent years, compared to their role ten to twenty years ago. Men and women who have recently become doctors are generally more amenable to pharmacist intervention and view them as an important healthcare resource.

Assertive Communication Skills

Assertive communication occurs when the individual expresses opinions directly and actions correlate with words. Assertive communicators are respectful of others and not bullying but firm and honest about opinions. They frequently use "I" statements to make their point: "I would like. . .". Communication usually includes cooperative statements, such as "What do you think?" and distinguishes between fact and opinion. Assertive communicators often engender trust in others because they are consistent, honest, and open in communicating with others. The assertive communicator feels free to express disagreement and anger but does so in a manner that is nonthreatening and respectful of others' feelings. Assertive communication requires a strong sense of self-worth and the belief that personal opinions have value. Assertive communicators tend to have good listening skills because they value the opinions of others and feel comfortable collaborating.

Aspects of a Leader

A **good leader** is necessary to run an efficient pharmacy that will both serve the needs of the patient's health and financial situation, while at the same time maintaining the financial needs of the healthcare and insurance companies. A leader is not the same thing as a manager, although a good manager is often also a good leader. A leader is someone who has a vision for improvement and can easily pull others toward this vision and lead the pharmacy into a new era. A good leader must have both a decent personal ethical system by which they always abide and a strong professional outlook toward pharmacy. A leader must have a strong vision and develop relationships with ease in order to pull people into that vision so that the vision will not be a simple idea, but can soon be turned into a reality. As a leader it is important to never stop learning and to continually adapt ideas as healthcare evolves, and finally it important to pass knowledge to future generations of leaders by mentoring these people so that they too can one day lead healthcare into the future.

Importance of Cultivating Relationships as a Leader

Developing strong relationships are one of the most important aspects of leadership. Without proper relationships, little will get done. A strong leader must adopt appropriate relationship skills with all aspects of the pharmacy, treating each and every person that works for them with kind firmness and respect. Additionally, relationships are needed outside the pharmacy as well, including with patients, as well as other healthcare colleagues. A strong leader with strong relationship skills can help connect all aspects of healthcare with the pharmacy.

STEPS TO PROBLEM SOLVING

Problem solving to anticipate or prevent recurrences of patient/family dissatisfaction involves arriving at a hypothesis, testing, and assessing the data to determine if the hypothesis holds true. If a problem has arisen, taking steps to resolve the immediate problem is only the first step if recurrence is to be avoided:

1. **Define the issue**: Talk with the patient or family and staff to determine if the problem is related to a failure of communication or other issues, such as culture or religion.
2. **Collect data**: This may mean interviewing additional staff or reviewing documentation, and gaining a variety of perspectives.
3. **Identify important concepts**: Determine if there are issues related to values or beliefs.
4. **Consider reasons for actions**: Distinguish between motivation and intention on the part of all parties to determine the reason for the problem.
5. **Make decision**: A decision on how to prevent a recurrence of a problem should be based on advocacy and moral agency, reaching the best solution possible for the patient, family, or staff.

HEALTH LITERACY

PATIENTS

Health literacy in its most basic form relates to a patient's ability to comprehend and utilize health resources. Health resources can include various health related services such as: health care in a clinic or hospital, receiving health information in the form of informational pamphlets, understanding information related to medication usage and education related managing chronic illnesses. In more specific terms, health literacy relates to a patient's ability to utilize and understand health resources within a specific cultural and social paradigm. Language and social barriers are the most common reasons a patient has low health literacy. Most healthcare and healthcare related information is in English and geared toward a general population that has lived in the United States for a long period of time and is familiar with the general framework of this healthcare system.

HEALTH CARE PROVIDERS

It is easy to assume that healthcare professionals have a high level of health literacy, but this is not always true. For **health care providers**, health literacy is focused on continuing education and cultural sensitivity. For health care providers to have continued good health literacy, it is vital that they keep up-to-date with current healthcare related research and clinical trials. This can be accomplished in several ways including: reading journal articles, being involved in journal clubs and grand rounds, attending local continuing education forums and good communication with peers. Continuing education related to cultural sensitivity involves further education related to the culture, religion and customs of the patient base being seen. It can also include learning how to speak relevant languages and specific education relating to various cultural beliefs and religions.

IMPROVING PATIENT HEALTH LITERACY

There are numerous ways that healthcare providers can **improve health literacy**. In general, providing culturally sensitive healthcare material and translating educational pamphlets into multiple languages will improve health literacy a great deal. Additionally, wording educational pamphlets in easier to understand terms will also improve health literacy. Staff education is also vital to improve patient health literacy. As clinic staff is often who a patient speaks and interacts with first, it is vital that staff is trained in cultural sensitivity. This way, patients are treated appropriately from the very beginning and are more likely to return for further healthcare. As a pharmacist, you can improve health literacy by translating medication information in the appropriate language and if possible, counsel in the appropriate language. It is also vital that important medication auxiliary labels are also translated into the appropriate language.

Cultural Competency

In the most general terms, cultural competency relates to the capacity for one person to perceive and understand another person's cultural beliefs. This is especially vital for healthcare professionals who encounter a variety of patients from a variety of cultural backgrounds. In the healthcare industry, cultural competency relates to the ability to not only find appropriate ways to communicate with patients from other cultures, but also to not discriminate or judge solely based on a patients cultural background. The best way to gain cultural competency is to learn about a variety of cultural customs and ask appropriate questions to your patients. Often, patients are very honest and love to explain their cultural views if asked in a non-judgmental way.

Communication with Patients

In the healthcare profession, communication is key. This is especially the case when you are working with patients that have a different cultural background. While not always the case, language barriers are a large part of working with a patient from a different cultural background. It is important to find a way to properly communicate with patients that do not speak English. Ideally, there is a bilingual medical professional available to translate. If this is not possible, there are many resources that can translate important medical information to the patient over the phone. In addition, most pharmacies have medication information in several different languages. This is not to be used as the only means of communicating with a patient who does not speak English, but used as a resource that a patient can use at home.

Biostatistics and Research Methods

Hypothesis Testing

Hypothesis testing is an important component in statistics that involves two opposite and conflicting hypotheses about a given data set. The concept of hypothesis testing surrounds the ideas that if one hypothesis is not correct, the other would be. For example, if the alternative hypothesis was that A would turn into X, then the null hypothesis would be that A does not turn into X. If the data collected significantly represents that A most certainly turns into X, then the alternative hypothesis will be accepted and the null hypothesis will be rejected. If the data does not support the alternative hypothesis, then the null hypothesis could not be rejected, indicating that results seen may not be of a significant difference and the alternative hypothesis was incorrect.

Independent and Dependent Variables

The **independent variable** is the variable in the experiment that is directly manipulated by the experimenter. The **dependent variable** is what is measured in an experiment in response to the independent variable. For example, an experiment involves measuring at various doses of amphotericin B and their effect on liver toxicity; the different doses of amphotericin B is the independent variable, as it is changed by the experimenter, while the severity of the liver toxicity is the dependent variable, measured in response to the changes in the amphotericin B dose.

Translational Research

Translational research is a relatively new approach to biomedical sciences. It combines the clinic and hospital with basic laboratory science. It usually involves going into hospitals and observing what is needed, e.g., observing patients of a particular disease state, including biopsies, and taking this information into the lab to guide research and create new possible therapies that can be taken and used again in the clinic as potential therapy. While this approach has always been the general underlying concept of biomedical sciences, it takes a more direct approach in research, allowing for less blind guessing in the quest for new therapies, and instead leading to a shorter research and development time for safer and more effective drugs.

Important Steps in Basic Experimental Design

Generally, any experiment starts out with a vague concept, an idea that wants to be tested. When this vague concept has been developed, a literature search should be done, such as in PubMed to see if this idea has any validity or if anyone has tested it yet. There is no purpose for doing an experiment if it's already been done. From this PubMed search, enough information should be garnered to create a more succinct idea or concept that will be tested. Additionally, an educated guess, a hypothesis, of what is expected to happen should be developed. After these initial parts of the experiment have been performed, several sets of experiments should be performed to prove the hypothesis. If the experiments are unable to prove the hypothesis as wrong, the hypothesis in relation to the experiment is considered as correct. Experiments should be repeated numerous times and statistics should be performed to determine significance.

Data Types

The following are various types of data:

- **Qualitative data**: Also known as categorical data, usually involves a non-numerical set of data, such as measuring emotions in the concept of being happy, sad or indifferent. The data represents a set of emotions, but are not quantifiable.
- **Quantitative data**: A numerical based measured data set. Types of quantitative data include discrete and continuous.
- **Discrete data**: Occurs if the measured values are finite and in distinct classes. An example of this is when a group of measurements are given numerical values, such as an opinions (agree-1/ disagree-2) in a survey or emotional states due to certain tests (happy-1/sad-2/angry-3/indifferent-4). Each subject will fall into one category with no overlap.
- **Continuous data**: Data that can be measured on a nearly infinite scale. There are no set categories of values. Examples of this can include: height, weight, length, or width.

Accuracy Versus Precision

Accuracy involves how close the measured data is to the "true" value. **Precision** involves how close replicated measurements are to each other. A measurement can be accurate, close to the true value, but not have great precision, thus lousy repeatability. Also, a measurement could be off from the "true" value, thus not accurate, although the repeated measurements could be close to each other, and thus very precise. Measured data can be all over the place, thus show little accuracy and little precision. Finally, if the values are close to the "true" value of the experiment, and the replicates are very close, the measurement would be both accurate and precise. In scientific research, accuracy is not important because the true value is not known, although precision is very important. When a "true" value is known, the bioavailability of a drug for example, then accuracy can become very important.

Type I and Type II Errors

A **type I error (α)** indicates a false positive, in which the null hypothesis was rejected, although it should not have been. A type I error is not wanted, because it can lead to false conclusions, which can prove fatal if it goes unnoticed during drug development. The probability of a type I error is generally recorded as a p-value of less than 0.05 or 0.01, which states that there is only a 5% or 1% chance of a type I error occurring in a specific experiment. This percentage is generally accepted as significantly different in experiments. A **type II error (β)** is known as a false negative, when the null hypothesis was not rejected, when it should have been. Type II errors are unwanted, as important findings could have gone undiscovered, which could have disastrous effects during drug development as well. Type II errors depend on statistical power of the experiment; as power of an experiment increases the probability of type II error occurring decreases. Power depends on significance level, sample size, and accuracy of the measurements.

Statistical Significance and Clinical Significance

Statistical significance deals mainly with population size and measures the probability of a certain outcome from occurring not from chance alone. While important in research, statistical significance may not have a strong bearing in the hospital or clinical setting. **Clinical significance** has little to do with statistics but more to do with judgment and feasibility of a certain treatment to be effective in treating a certain population. If a hospital needs to treat another hundred people to get a significant difference in a population, the clinical effects are not considered significant. In other words, statistics lies in the realm of probability and mathematics, while clinical significance lies in the real world.

Student's T-Test

Students T-test is a statistical test that analyzes the significance of two different groups. Often the groups are an experimental population compared to a control population. The T-test must have some assumptions to work including a normal distribution of the data and equal variance. The samples can be dependent or independent. Dependent T-tests are used when the samples that are tested are the same, such as in the case of replicates. Independent T-tests can be used to measure two different groups of data if the population size (n) is equal between the two groups. If the sample size is different, variable calculations are used.

Normal and Binomial Distribution

Normal distributions are sometimes known as bell-curves and generally have an equal distribution of data and point closer to the means. The shape of a normal distribution can change due to differences in the standard deviation and the mean. **Binomial distribution** is a statistical model that measures the distribution of data that is considered mutually exclusive; it is either one or the other. For example, a flip of the coin can only be heads or tails, not both. A person is either experiencing an adverse effect of a drug or they are not. Binomial distributions must assume that outcomes are independent, mutually exclusive, randomly selected and fall into one of two categories.

Kurtosis and Skewness

Kurtosis is a statistical measurement that describes the peak of a statistical distribution, which usually differs from highly peaked to flat distribution. Kurtosis examines and measures the level of distribution of data around the mean of the population. **Skewness** measures the level of symmetry around the center-point or mean of a distribution. There are negative and positive measurements of skewness. Negative skewness occurs when most of the data is right of what is observed in a normal distribution. Positive skewness occurs when most of the data is left of what is observed in a normal distribution.

External Validity and Internal Validity

External validity relates to how well results from a study (clinical trial) can be generalized to a larger population. If the results of a study are shown to extrapolate to a larger population is it thought to have a high external validity; on the flip-side, if the results cannot be generalized to a larger population, the study is thought to have a low external validity. **Internal validity** involves determining a cause and effect relationship between two variables such as drug X leads to disorder Y. The stronger the relationship and the more alternative cause/effect relationships can be ignored, then the higher the internal validity of the experiment. An experiment with low internal validity would show little to no cause/effect relationship between two variables, or it would show many possible alternative cause/effect relationships.

Possible Abuses of Statistics

There are many ways **statistics can be abused and misused**, giving a false representation of the data. For example, graphing data but altering axis values in order to misrepresent data significance, even though technically correct, the visual data changes would seem larger or smaller than the actual truth. Additionally, a small sample size could provide false positives or false negatives, as it may not be a large enough representation of the entire population. Misuse of statistical tests is also another way that statistics are often abused; often appearing that the null hypothesis was rejected and the observed changes in the data set were significant even though this was not true. Statistics can also be abused due to loaded questions as well as missing and distorted data.

Social and Behavioral Aspects of Pharmacy Practice

Importance of Customer Service in a Pharmacy

The patients' health should be the pharmacist's utmost priority; however, as a business and in the eyes of a customer, **customer service** is one of the most important components. Without proper customer service, a patient/customer will quickly go to another pharmacy. If customer service is incredible, many customers will look past higher prices, thus increasing the profit potential of the pharmacy. Treat each patient with respect, never with rudeness or arrogance. Express empathy, an understanding of what the patient is going through. If the patient asks questions answer them with a smile. If mistakes are made, fix them quickly without argument. If complaints are made by a customer, see to them and rectify them as quickly as possible. If a complaint is observed, respected and fixed, most customers will return for repeat business. If not, customers will most likely tell many more people about the awful service they had received from your business, thus causing the pharmacy to lose more customers

Behavior Toward Healthcare

The types of behavior toward healthcare as described by the health brief model are described below:

- **Health behavior**: Someone who views themselves as being healthy and takes several preventative methods to keep themselves healthy including dieting, exercise, therapy, routine visits to the doctors' office, routine checking for signs of breast cancer or testicle cancer.

- **Illness behavior**: Someone who views themselves as possibly being ill or becoming ill, and their behavior will relate to this, including going to see a doctor, talk about healthcare issues with loved ones and pharmacists, take unnecessary over-the-counter drugs (experimenting with over-the counter drugs).
- **Sick-role behavior**: Someone who, based on a diagnosis by a doctor and based on these findings, will adhere to the medical diagnosis, prescribed drug regimen, using over-the-counter drugs that as suggested by a doctor or pharmacists, getting plenty of rest, and taking plenty of time to recuperate.

Patient Misconceptions of Retail Pharmacy

Only recently have patients begun to trust pharmacists; however, this trust is limited. Often patients only see pharmacists in a retail setting and really do not grasp the role a pharmacist has in healthcare. This is partially due to the **patients' misconceptions**; they see that a pharmacist puts drugs in a bottle and nothing else. In the patients' eyes, a pharmacist has a reasonably simple job. On the flip-side pharmacists have not done much to contradict these misconceptions until recently. Pharmacists often do not deal with patients as much, they approach patients coldly, and unfortunately many pharmacist, particularly in the retail setting, simply do not treat patients with respect either. Respect must be given both ways. Additionally, the way companies advertise pharmacies, with drive-thru windows, with the promise of one hour prescription filling (which often is not met), patients often do not view pharmacies with much higher regard then they do a fast-food restaurant. These misconceptions can be changed, if the pharmacist desires to change them.

Patient Misconceptions of Hospital Pharmacists

In a **hospital setting**, pharmacists are often invisible. Healthcare is a team effort, however, ingrained notions of medical doctors being the sole providers of healthcare has tainted patients' views. Additionally, pharmacists often do not get to know their patients as readily as other healthcare providers and often go unnoticed. Also, patients often don't trust pharmacists in relation to other healthcare providers. A patient will often not trust a pharmacist to give them immunizations, or they would feel uncomfortable, although this comfort level is higher in a hospital setting (mainly because many patients don't realize that the person administering the injection is a pharmacist) than retail settings. As a pharmacist it is essential that the patients' trust is gained, and to do this, it is important that the pharmacist talks to the patient as a person and does not simply focus on lab values.

Potential Drug Seeking Behavior

As a pharmacist it is important to be respectful and trusting of patients; if this is done, they too will respect and trust you. However, as a pharmacist you must also be adept in spotting **drug-seeking behavior** which is often a sign of drug addiction, often of opioids or other pain medication. Possible warning signs may include: multiple prescriptions for multiple drugs of the same class of prescriptions from multiple doctors from multiple clinics, forged prescriptions, multiple prescriptions filled at multiple pharmacies and inappropriate prescribed drug number for disease state. All of these situations will often come with a story or explanation or excuse from the patient. While these are possible red flags of drug-seeking behavior, they are not sure signs, and any suspicions should be investigated further before accusing a patient. Call the doctor about the prescriptions, call other pharmacies, etc.

Behavior Modification

Behavior modification is a type of systematic therapy that works toward the goal of replacing maladaptive behaviors with positive behaviors. This type of therapy can be utilized with individuals, groups or entire communities. There are 3 types of behavioral modification:

- **Operant conditioning** utilizes positive reinforcement directed towards the desired behaviors. By utilizing positive reinforcement, the participant will want to repeat the good behaviors to gain the reward, creating a new pattern of Operant conditioning can be effective with eating disorders, smoking cessation, or addictions.
- **Desensitization** in which clients are increasingly exposed to those things that cause them stress (such as phobias) so that they can overcome their fears.
- **Aversion therapy** applies a negative consequence to an action (such as using medications to induce vomiting after drinking alcohol) to create negative associations with the action in order to modify behavior.

Role of Pharmacist in Caregiving Throughout the Life Cycle

The role of the pharmacist throughout the **life cycle** incudes:

- **Embryonic and fetal development**: Monitor drugs for potential teratogenic effects and pregnancy category in order to provide information to patients and healthcare providers.
- **Neonatal period**: Titrate drugs for size and developmental stage, compound drugs as needed, recommend vaccinations, and evaluate response to drug therapy.
- **Infancy**: Similar to neonatal period but must be aware of changes in the child's development and must be alert to medications that carry specific pediatric warnings, such as those that may affect development of bones or teeth.
- **Childhood**: Similar to infancy. Know dosing ranges for common drugs and titrate drugs according to age and size, educate patient/family, and provide expertise to other healthcare providers.
- **Adulthood**: Educate patients regarding drug-drug reactions, toxicity, and adverse effects, recommend disease preventive therapies, and discuss birth control options.
- **Older adulthood**: Understand differences in absorption, distribution, metabolism, and elimination of drugs related to age and provide guidance regarding treatment for chronic and acute illness.

Adherence

Adherence (compliance) refers to a patient's ability to adhere to a specific diagnosed drug regimen as suggested by the doctor or pharmacist. Improper drug adherence can cause many healthcare issues including an ineffective treatment of the patient's disease. Poor adherence can also lead to societal healthcare issues, such as improper use of antibiotics has led to the formation of more resistant bacterial strains. Errors in adherence can be due to many reasons, including forgetfulness, the purpose of the treatment not being clarified properly to the patient and the patient being too embarrassed to ask questions, lack of effect perceived or otherwise, side effects real or imagined, or the patient started to feel better and felt that taking the remainder of the drug was unnecessary. Ways to improve adherence include more effective counseling on drug regimens. Make sure patients understand the course of treatment and the importance of following this treatment until finished, unless due to awful side effects. Ultimately however, it is the patient's choice to adhere or not to a drug regimen and they will do as they please.

Role of Pharmacist in Death and Dying with Dignity

The role of the pharmacist in **death and dying** with dignity includes:

- **Serving as a resource person/educating patient and family**: The pharmacist may provide information about medications, drug-drug interactions, and adverse effects as well as alternative drugs or complementary therapies that may provide comfort. Patients with nausea, vomiting, and/or anorexia may need guidance regarding supplements and treatments available.
- **Being knowledgeable about analgesia**: The pharmacist should have a broad understanding of the different types of analgesia and approaches to pain control, especially for those with severe and/or intractable pain. Additionally, the pharmacist must be aware of concerns about addiction and habituation and educate healthcare providers, patients, and family accordingly.
- **Referral to hospice**: If the pharmacist is aware that a patient has a life-threatening disease then the pharmacist may be in a position to refer a patient/family to hospice care and provide information about services they provide, such as helping control pain.

Medication Dispensing and Distribution Systems

Models of Medication Distribution in Hospitals

There are three chief **models for medication distribution** in hospitals: centralized, decentralized, and hybrid.

- The **centralized distribution** is typical of most traditional hospitals: a single pharmacy is in charge of filling all orders required by the practitioners and sending them to the proper nursing stations for administration.
- The **decentralized distribution** uses multiple housing stations for medications, e.g. automated dispensing cabinets (ADCs); a single pharmacy is again in charge of processing practitioner orders, but the medications are released to nurses by the housing stations.
- The **hybrid case** combines both models, usually specific to each case of medication or strength.

Other variations of medication distribution include: satellite pharmacies, which consist of smaller pharmacies with limited resources spread throughout the hospital; bulk distribution of medication to nurse stations rather than single-dose distribution; robots in stations similar to ADCs which fill required variable orders; pneumatic tubes (usually with PIN or ID locks) which range throughout the hospital from a pharmacy to areas of interest; and mobile carts which may move throughout the hospital and nursing areas.

Medication-Use Systems

Adverse drug events (ADEs) are accidents which can, in a worst-case scenario, result in the wrong dosage of the wrong medication being delivered in the wrong manner to the wrong patient. To combat this, hospitals and pharmacies may institute plans, training, or 'systems' to address weak links in the medication administration pathway, including prescription of the drug itself, its dispensation, or administration. That is, **"medication-use systems"** is a broad term which encompasses any system that helps to guard against ADEs. To help ensure proper prescription, medication-use systems might emphasize attention to patient demographic and clinical information or the drug information. In some cases, the wrong medication is given to the consumer; here, a system might recognize the importance of proper communication of drug information between hospital and pharmacy staffs or better methods of drug labeling, packaging, storage, or distribution. To protect from drugs being administered improperly, some plans may focus on the education of staff and patients who handle and administer the drugs. Medication-use systems may also suggest higher standards of staff competency or increased quality and risk assessment /management.

High Alert Medications

High alert medications, such as digoxin, are drugs that generally have a narrow therapeutic range and have a high potential to cause patient harm if they are not properly prescribed and dispensed. High alert medications do not necessarily have a higher rate of medication error and near miss medication error, but the potential for patient harm is much greater with these drugs if a medication error does occur. Most hospital and retail pharmacy computer programs flag specific medications as high alert medications and require that the pharmacist double check the written prescription and dose. Some programs even require a second pharmacist to double the check the first pharmacist. It is important that, as a pharmacist, you do not undermine these double checks in your computer system. They are there to protect the patient and the patient is always your priority.

Role of Pharmacy Informatics and Information Management

Pharmacy informatics relates to data regarding medications and knowledge about the healthcare system and how drugs are acquired, stored, disseminated, and administered. Information management includes knowledge of CPOE systems and clinical decision software systems as well as electronic prescriptions, barcoding, electronic medication administration records, inventory systems (automated and manual), and equipment, such as automated medication dispensing carts and smart pumps. Management also includes an understanding of pharmacy metrics and the ability to manage, analyze, and report data (qualitative, quantitative, primary, and secondary). Management requires awareness of the 4 types of healthcare data: medical/clinical (patient-specific from medical records), knowledge-based (research, education), comparison (internal or external), and aggregate (includes pharmacy transactions) and how these are expressed in pharmacy informatics. Information management also includes knowledge of data representation (binary code, hexadecimal code, Uni-code standard), data aggregation, and statistical measures, such as measure of averages and distribution.

iPLEDGE

iPLEDGE is a risk management computer program which was developed to decrease the potential teratogenic effect of Accutane (isotretinoin) on unborn fetuses. Approved by the FDA, it requires that all healthcare personnel (physicians and pharmacists), all wholesale distributors and all patients prescribed isotretinoin, must be registered with iPLEDGE. Before a patient is given their prescription each month, they must be counseled of certain risks and must also meet certain criteria. Women have additional criteria that they must pass including two pregnancy tests with negative results before they are given their first prescription of isotretinoin and they must pass an additional pregnancy test each subsequent month before their prescription is refilled. Furthermore, it is suggested that women should use two birth control methods such as condoms and birth control pills, if sexually active while on the drug.

FMEA

Failure mode and effects analysis (FMEA) is used to better understand what type and frequency of medications errors. A FMEA involves forming a committee and/or using specialized computer programs to look at near miss medication errors and to evaluate potential holes in existing computer technology. The goal of a FMEA is to flag areas that could be contributing to medication errors and to develop techniques or alter computer technology in such a way that medication errors are significantly reduced. A FMEA can especially be beneficial in a hospital setting where a single computer system is being used by many different healthcare personnel.

Medication Errors

Medication errors include any and all avoidable incidents that allow the possibility of inappropriate medication use or harm to the patient while the medication is in the control of the administrator. Not all 'medication errors' necessarily end with real harm to the patient: the term also includes any actions which (though prevented) could have resulted in harm or wrongful use of medications. Medication errors can be due to miscommunication, such as poor handwriting or inaccurate information requests, confusion of similar drug names or dosing units, or improper amounts or directions supplied to the administrator. They may also include improper labeling, packaging, compounding, monitoring, and use of the medication itself. The most important response to medication errors (besides their correction) is to properly report them to prevent future incidents. Medication errors are initially reported to MedWatch before being reviewed by a branch of the FDA, the Department of Medication Error Prevention and Analysis (DMEPA), where causality and circumstances are analyzed to provide recommendations for future similar cases.

Medication Errors That Can Occur During Drug Point of Entry

Point of entry (POE) relates specifically to when a prescription or a drug order set is being prescribed by the physician. It is important to remember that physicians will often give a verbal drug order to the pharmacist, nurse or other healthcare professional. Misheard information from a verbal order is a common area where a medication error can occur. Always read back the medication order to the physician to confirm the verbal order was taken correctly. POE errors can also occur when the physician is distracted and accidently picks the wrong medication, dose or strength. POE errors can also occur when a physician writes a prescription that is illegible or is missing information. It is very important to call a physician and verify any information that is in anyway ambiguous. It is interesting to note that the use of computers during the initial order entry process can reduce medication errors by up to 50%.

Medication Errors That Can Occur During Drug Dispensing

In a retail pharmacy setting, **dispensing drug** relates to the action of physically filling and checking a prescription before it is given to a patient. In a hospital setting, drug dispensing can be more complicated. In this situation, medications may get filled and sent directly to the patient, or the medication may go to a Pyxis type machine where a nurse retrieves the drug based on a timed medication record (MAR). Medication errors related to drug dispensing can occur any time between the initial medication fill to right before the patient takes the medication. As a pharmacist, it is important to double check medication orders for patients before they are officially entered into the computer system. In a hospital setting, it is also important to check a new medication order against the current MAR. This can help you discover patient specific medication errors.

Medication Errors That Can Occur During Drug Administration

Medication errors related to **drug administration** can occur in hospital and outpatient settings. Common hospital related administration medication errors include improper administration method (giving an IM shot subcutaneously), giving the medication at the wrong time, giving the wrong amount, setting improper IV infusion rates or even giving the medication to the wrong patient. Retail related administration medication errors include dispensing the wrong medication to the patient, improper directions on the medication label and the patient misinterpreting medication instructions. Drug administration medication errors can be avoided in both settings by checking and re-checking medication orders and routes of administration. In a retail setting, it is important to make sure the right prescription gets to the right patient. Always verify that you are handing the correct prescription bottle to the correct patient.

Drugs That Either Sound Alike or Look Alike

Drugs that have similar names, that sound alike when spoken or look alike on a shelf are often drugs involved in medication errors. Always double check medications that could be mistaken for another medication to make sure the correct medication is dispensed. The following is a list of some medications that are common **sound alike or look alike** medication error culprits:

- Fosamax and Flomax
- Prilosec and Prozac
- Celebrex and Cerebyx
- Zantac and Zerit and Zyrtec
- Metadate and Methadone
- Depakote and Depakene and Depacon
- Taxol and Taxotere
- Keppra and Kaletra
- Narcan and Norcuron
- Lamictal and Lamisil
- Serzone and Seroquel
- Reminyl and Amaryl

Abbreviations

In the fast paced medical world, it is not surprising that almost every medical term or instruction can be abbreviated in some way. While **abbreviations** will always be a part of the medical vernacular, it is important to recognize that abbreviations can be easily mistaken and misunderstood. Always double check any abbreviation that could potentially mean more than one drug or instruction. Below is a very brief list of common abbreviations that can be interpreted multiple ways:

- QD, means daily. Interpreted as QOD, write daily instead.
- SC or SQ, means subcutaneously. Interpreted as SL, spell specific route instead.
- Per OS, means orally. Interpreted as OS or OU, write orally instead.
- TIW, means thrice weekly. Interpreted as TID, spell out three times weekly.
- D/C, means dispense at discharge. Interpreted as discontinue medication, spell out instead.
- Ug, means micrograms. Interpreted as mg, spell out instead.
- AU, AS, AD, means ear. Interpreted as OU, OS, always check route.

Medication Error Statistics

While **statistics related to medication errors** always change, it is important to have a good general knowledge of medication error rates. Always remember that the goal of a pharmacist is to be as error free as possible. Below is a list of recent statistics related to medication error rates.

- Medication errors have been attributed to over 7,000 deaths a year.
- At least 30% of patients receiving medical care in a hospital have been subjected to a medication error.
- The most common medication error in a hospital setting is a medical error related to drug administration.

- Medication errors cost hospitals millions of dollars each year.
- The medication error rate in ambulatory and retail setting is over 25%.

Dealing with Pharmacy Mistakes

While working for as well as managing a pharmacy, it is important to realize **medical errors** will occur. As a pharmacy manager, it is important to treat all medical errors seriously, but with an understanding that people, machines, and general systems of operations, make mistakes. Nothing is foolproof. Mistakes should be talked about and dealt with calmly and with understanding. In a positive environment like this, people are far more likely to fix errors rather than ignore them. Records should be kept of errors that occur, not as a form of punishment, but as a means to measure frequency of errors and determine how to fix these mistakes in the future. When dealing with patients' complaints; be understanding, polite, and if reasonable fix the error as soon as possible. Patients view mistakes harshly, because it is their health, real or perceived, that is at stake.

Pharmacist's Role in Reducing Medical Errors

Physicians, pharmacists, nurses, and other healthcare staff make mistakes, unfortunately medical errors lead to numerous deaths in the US. These can be contributed to misdiagnosis, poor patient history, development of allergies, miscommunication of a therapy, drug-drug interactions, etc. **Pharmacists** are the last resource before a drug therapy reaches the patient, and as a pharmacist, it is vital for them to learn how to minimize medical errors. These can include being very careful in distributing the correct drug to the correct patient. It is also important for the pharmacist to have knowledge of other prescriptions the patient may be on, in order to decrease chances of undesired drug-drug interactions. A pharmacist must be willing to question a prescription or a diagnosis by a physician, if a possible mistake has been made. Additionally, another way to reduce medical errors, as a pharmacist, is to clearly counsel patients on their prescriptions, making sure they understand the instructions for their medicine.

Attempts by the Healthcare Community to Reduce Medical Errors

In order to reduce confusion of similarly sounding names of drugs, the **FDA regulates the brand names** that pharmaceutical companies are allowed to use, decreasing the likelihood of one or more drugs sounding similar and thus decreasing the chance of miss-prescribing. Also, more hospitals and pharmacies are adopting a barcode approach to regulating drugs. A barcode is on the drug and the patient. Before the drug is administered, the patient and the drug are scanned to make sure the drug, and dose of the drug are correct for the correct patient. Additionally, a law was recently passed to make it illegal for prescriptions to be written in cursive. Instead they must be clearly printed by hand or printed by a computer to decrease chances of confusion about the prescription.

Monitoring by the FDA of Hospitals and Pharmacies for Medication Errors

While the FDA does not have a formal drug medication error monitoring system, they do keep a watchful eye on medication error rates in hospitals and retail pharmacies across the United States. The FDA accomplishes this by compiling and monitoring information that is passed on to them via the **United States Pharmacopeia (USP**) and the **Institute for Safe Medication Practices (ISMP).** By compiling data that is collected by several agencies, the FDA is able to gain a good perspective on the types of medication errors that are occurring in hospitals and pharmacies. Additionally, the FDA monitors adverse drug event information that is entered by healthcare professionals on their website, MedWatch. MedWatch is voluntary and anonymous and is extremely valuable, especially as it relates to drugs that are new to the market that may have adverse reactions that were not originally found in clinical trials.

Important Terms

Sample: A subset of the population that has been chosen for further data analysis, in hopes of inferences of the larger population (i.e., if you wanted to study human red-headed children, human red-headed children are a subset of a larger population of children, which in itself is a subset of a larger populations of humans as a whole).

Population: The population describes the entire class of variables in which usually a smaller subset of samples is chosen for further study (i.e. red-headed children)

Parameter: A characteristic or value of an entire population (i.e. red-hair).

Statistic: A measurable, often originally unknown characteristic of a given sample.

Mean: Also known as the average, in which the sum of the data set is divided by the sample size of the data set.

Mode: Describes a certain value within a data set population that occurs the most frequently.

Median: The value that lies in the middle of the observed distribution of the data points, in which an equal number of data points possess a value larger and smaller than the median value. Sometimes the same as the mean, but not always true.

Midrange: Also known as range, it is the mean between the largest and smallest values of a given set of data points.

Standard Deviation: Indicates the amount/frequency of variability of a data set away from the mean of the data set.

Adverse Drug Event (ADE): Relates to any event that occurs when a drug is being used at standard dosing and something happens that was not expected or wanted. ADE's typically require that the drug be stopped or the dosage changed and can potentially require additional supportive care and hospitalization. ADE's can be related to unexpected or unwanted reactions to medication and/or mistakes in administration of the drug.

Adverse Drug Reaction (ADR): Relates specifically to an event where a patient takes a medication at standard human dosing and has a reaction that causes an unwanted reaction. This can be related to any type of medication administration mistake or can be an unexpected allergic reaction to a medication that had previously not caused a reaction.

Side Effects (SE): Relates to medication induced reactions. These are often known reactions and include common drug reactions such as stomach ache, vomiting and rash.

Potential Adverse Drug Event (PADE): Relates to any medication dispensing error that could possibly harm a patient.

Maximum Allowable Costs (MAC): Maximum cost for a specific drug or other product paid for by a patient to a pharmacy.

Actual Acquisition Cost (AAC): The price that a pharmacy will pay for drugs and other items, before they sell them to patients and other consumers.

Average Wholesale Price (AWP): A published list of drug products.

Estimated Acquisition Cost (EAC): An estimate of drugs paid for by a pharmacy. Often used by Medicaid in reimbursement planning.

Capitation: When pharmacies are given a portion of money a month to take care of all prescriptions and services for patients belonging to a certain healthcare plan.

Coinsurance: Patients pay for a percentage of their healthcare as determined by the health insurance plan.

Copayment: Patients pay a fixed amount of money for healthcare services, rather than a percentage, as determined by the healthcare insurance plan.

Deductible: Patient pays a certain amount of their healthcare, before insurance company pays for remaining benefits.

Pharmacy Practice and Clinical Sciences

Clinical Pathophysiology

General Classes of Diseases

These categories are generalizations, and diseases can easily fall under one or more **category types**.

- **Infectious diseases**: Caused by foreign microbial agents such as bacteria, fungi, and viruses.
- **Allergic/autoimmune disorders**: Caused by hypersensitivity reactions (I, II, III, IV) of the immune system; can lead to disorders such as asthma, allergic rhinitis, and arthritis.
- **Metabolic disorders**: Caused by errors in the metabolic pathways; can lead to some serious health problems. An example of this can be seen with people who suffer from phenylketonuria (PKU) and cannot metabolize phenylalanine. Metabolic disorders can be caused by important dietary deficiencies, genetically inherited, or be symptoms of other underlying diseases.
- **Neoplastic disorders**: Caused by numerous environmental and genetic insults, leading to uncontrolled growth of tissue, leading to the development of tumors.
- **Toxic disorders**: Caused by toxins and toxicants to the body. An example of this could be cirrhosis of the liver in response to chronic ethanol consumption.
- **Psychiatric disorders**: Described as chemical imbalances; deals with alterations in brain signaling, such as changes in dopamine levels, which can lead to various mental disorders, including depression and schizophrenia.

Tumors

Defined below are several types of tumors:

- **Carcinoma**: Generally, the most common types of cancer by which malignant tumors form in epithelial cells of the organ tissue.
- **Lymphoma/leukemia**: Malignant tumors that develop from leukocytes, blood and bone marrow cells.
- **Sarcoma**: Occurs due to tumors developing in connective and supportive tissues, including the bone, muscle, blood vessels, adipose tissue, and soft tissue (tissue that surrounds and supports the internal organs).
- **Mesothelioma**: Specific tumors derived from the protective membrane lining (mesothelia) of organs, most commonly found in the outer-linings of the chest cavity and lungs, but could be found in the abdomen as well.
- **Glioma**: Tumors that form from abundant neuronal cells of the central nervous system known as glia.
- **Germinoma**: Tumors of the germ (reproductive) cells found in the ovaries and testis.
- **Choriocarcinoma**: An aggressive type of malignant cancer that originally forms in the placenta

Tumor Grade

Tumor grade is a system to classify neoplastic cells by how abnormal the cells appear beneath a microscope compared to normal tissue. Generally performed after a biopsy of a tumor, the tissue is given to a pathologist to study, who determines if the tumor is benign or malignant. The pathologist will also determine the degree of malignancy, by grading the cancer cells. Well-differentiated cells have an appearance that is close to that of normal tissue, while poor or undifferentiated cells have little to no discernable features that are similar to normal tissue. There are five stages of grading:

- Gx- grade cannot be determined.
- G1- well-differentiated tumor.
- G2-moderately differentiated tumor.
- G3-poorly differentiated tumor.
- G4-undifferentiated tumors.

G1 represents a low grade tumor, G2 represents an intermediate grade tumor, G3 and G4 represent a high grade tumor. Higher tumor grade and poorer differentiation often correlates to increased cancer aggression.

Stages of Tumor Progression

The stages of tumor progression are as follows:

1. The first stage involves cells that have bypassed normal growth restraints, leading to increased proliferation of cells as well as decreased apoptosis. This stage is known as **dysplasia**.
2. As growth continues unheeded, the amounts of mutations increase, due to the lack of the proper checks and balances necessary in cellular growth. The cells and tissues become oddly shaped, and show an apparent difference compared to normal cells. This stage is known as **hyperplasia**.
3. As the cells continue to grow, they develop **pre-invasive primary tumors**, such as carcinomas, in which the cells are encapsulated within the tumor. As the cancer progresses, cells begin to escape from the tumor, by invading into surrounding tissue as well as blood vessels, giving rise to metastases.
4. As **invasive cells** of the primary tumor reach the blood, they can reach distant organ sites, creating secondary tumors, inhibiting the function of important organ systems. It is the development of these secondary tumors that often lead to increased patient mortality.

Proto-Oncogene, Oncogene, and Tumor Suppressor

A **proto-oncogene** is a gene that during cancer progression has a high likelihood of becoming an oncogene, a gene that becomes expressed and or overtly active greater than normal in response to mutation or changes in cellular signaling. **Oncogenes** are one component necessary for cells to bypass normal host restraints that govern proliferation, apoptosis, and migration, allowing tumors to grow and cancers to thrive. An example of an oncogene is Ras, a small protein that regulates essential cellular pathways. Up-regulating Ras can transform some normal cells into malignant cancer cells. **Tumor suppressor** is a gene or protein that is generally lost during the cancer progression. Tumor suppressors, if transfected and expressed at high levels in a cancer cell, will generally retard growth, increase cell death, and decrease migration. Tumor suppressors are lost for many reasons, including genetic mutations as well as epigenetic factors, such as increased methylation of the gene promoter, which would inhibit transcription of the gene. A prime example of a tumor suppressor is p53.

Diabetes Insipidus, Cretinism, and Goiter

The causes, symptoms, and treatments for diabetes insipidus, cretinism, and goiter are explained below:

- **Diabetes insipidus**: A disorder that leads to excessive thirst and loss of fluids through dilute urine. It is largely caused by a deficiency/decrease in vasopressin secretion in response to some injury to the pituitary gland (i.e. tumor growth). Treatment includes regulation of fluids, prevention of dehydration. Synthetic vasopressin or drugs that induce vasopressin (i.e. Chlorpropamide) can be given as a treatment.
- **Cretinism (congenital hypothyroidism):** A disorder in children due to decreased levels of thyroid hormones, that if left untreated can lead to stunted growth and severe intellectual disability. Treatable if caught in time by providing thyroxine to the patient.
- **Goiter**: An enlargement of the thyroid gland, often a symptom of more serious disease of the thyroid. Goiter can be caused by low iodine in the diet, or a sign of Grave's disease, in which the thyroid is hyper active. An unusual growth in the neck is a common sign of a goiter. Treatment often includes surgical removal of the thyroid, in part or totally, and hormone replacement therapy.

Acute Kidney Injury

Acute kidney injury **(AKI)** is described as rapid loss of function of kidneys, which can lead to an increase or urea build-up, a shift in the acid-base homeostasis, and a shift in electrolyte balances. Symptoms include altered levels of urination, hypovolemia, hypotension, rapid heart rate, edema, shortness of breath and it can also lead to hypertension, altered levels of electrolytes, etc. AKI can be subdivided into Prerenal, Intrinsic, or Postrenal. Prerenal AKI is often caused by lower blood perfusion into the kidneys, leading to a lower ability of kidneys to filter the blood properly. It can be caused by numerous disorders such as dehydration or liver cancer, and certain drugs can induce this disorder. Intrinsic AKI is caused by damage of the kidneys, which can be caused by inflammation, blood clots in the renal system, etc. Postrenal AKI can be caused by any obstruction of urine flow from the kidneys. This can be caused by kidney stones, an enlarged prostate, bladder cancer, etc.

Chronic Kidney Disease

Chronic kidney disease **(CKD)** is diagnosed in someone who has less than a glomerular filtration rate (GFR) of 60 mL/min per area of 1.73 m^2 for at least three months or has evidence of kidney damage for at least three months (albuminuria, structural changes, or abnormal urine sediment). It is generally caused by kidney damage secondary to diabetes, hypertension, or chronic infection.

- Patients with **Stage I CKD** have kidney damage with normal GFR ($\geq$90).
- Patients with **Stage II CKD** have kidney damage and slightly decreased GFR levels (60–89).
- Patients with **Stage III CKD** suffer from kidney damage and intermediately decreased GFR levels (30–59).
- In **Stage IV CKD**, patients suffer from a severe decrease in GFR level (15–29) in response to kidney damage.
- During **Stage V CKD**, patients are in kidney failure and have a GFR level of <15.

Symptoms include foaming of urine due to higher levels of albumin, either microalbuminuria (albumin levels 30–300 mg/day) or albuminuria (levels of albumin in urine exceed 300 mg/day). Other symptoms include hypertension, edema, and anemia.

Acute Organ Rejection

Acute rejection of a transplanted organ is a major problem with solid organ transplants. During the transplantation, the patient that is receiving the organ is immediately exposed to antigens from the donor organ. The immune system of the organ recipient does not recognize the antigens of the new organ, and an immune response occurs, leading to rejection of the transplanted organ. While unpleasant and not desired, it is a normal response of the body to foreign tissue. Many important factors can increase the chance for acute rejection of an organ including mismatched HLA between organ donor and organ recipient. Acute rejection may be higher in children for certain organs and can be higher with previous organ rejection, pregnancy, or if an organ was taken from a deceased donor. Immunosuppressive drugs are used to lower the chance of acute rejection. A drug regimen of immunosuppressants must be individualized and an important balance must be struck. The use of immunosuppressants must be enough to treat rejection of the organ, but not too much that unwarranted infections occur and toxicity is kept at a minimum.

Review Video: Immunomodulators and Immunosuppressive Agents
Visit mometrix.com/academy and enter code: 666131

Respiratory Alkalosis and Respiratory Acidosis

Respiratory alkalosis is caused by hyperventilation, which leads to excessive CO_2 excretion from the lungs. This leads to decreased plasma levels of CO_2 and increased pH. Respiratory alkalosis is often associated with increased anxiety and can also be caused by going from a low altitude to a high altitude where there is less available oxygen in the environment, resulting in a prolonged increased respiratory rate. Changes in pressure can lead to increased CO_2 ventilation. Symptoms include rapid uncontrollable breathing. It can also lead to numbness as well as a tingling sensation in the skin. Treatment requires addressing the underlying cause to calm the individual, decrease respiratory rate, and increase the likelihood of re-breathing in CO_2 and returning the pH to normal. **Respiratory acidosis** occurs in response to decreased CO_2 excretion. Plasma CO_2 levels are increased as well as levels of carbonic acid, leading to a decrease in pH levels. Compensation can include increased bicarbonate formation. Symptoms include shortness of breath, dizziness, and confusion. Treatment can include oxygen replacement and the use of bronchodilators to open airway passages if, for example, the underlying cause is asthma. Often respiratory alkalosis is a symptom of an underlying disorder.

Metabolic Alkalosis and Metabolic Acidosis

Metabolic alkalosis occurs in response to lower levels of hydrogen ions in the blood. It is commonly associated with uncontrolled vomiting, which can lead to increased level of bicarbonate in the body, increasing pH. The body undergoes hypoventilation in order to attempt to return pH levels back to normal. Increased excretion of bicarbonate by the kidneys can also help in returning pH levels back to normal. Symptoms include slow deep breathing as well as periods of apnea or lack of breathing. If untreated it can lead to irregular heart rhythm, nausea, and irritability. Treatment can include addition of saline solution by IV. **Metabolic acidosis** occurs in response to an increased level of hydrogen ions in the blood. This can be caused by increased production of hydrogen atoms as well as decreased ability of kidneys to form bicarbonate, a necessary sequestration agent of hydrogen ions in the body. Symptoms include shallow breathing, headaches, and lack of energy. Treatment includes replacement of fluids and electrolytes, dialysis if due to kidney failure, or replacement by sodium bicarbonate.

Vitamin Deficiencies

Vitamins A, C, and E

Symptoms of **vitamin A deficiency** include dry inflamed eyes, dry skin, and decreased night vision. It can also lead to increased susceptibility to respiratory infections and can decreased growth in children. **Vitamin C deficiency** symptoms include increased nose bleeding, weakness and fatigue if mild. If severe, deficiency can lead to scurvy, which can lead to excessive bleeding, severely swollen gums, and poor healing. **Vitamin E deficiency** is rare. Symptoms include anemia, decreased coordination, muscle weakness, inability to feel position of limbs in relationship to torso. Vitamin A deficiency can also lead to massive brain hemorrhaging in infants.

Vitamins B1, B2, B3, and B5

Vitamin B1, B2, B3, and B5 deficiencies are as follows:

- **Vitamin B1 (thiamine)**: Deficiencies can lead to beriberi (a disorder of the nervous system) emotional problems, weakness and fatigue. Thiamine deficiencies can also lead to cardiac arrest if severe enough.
- **Vitamin B2 (riboflavin)**: Deficiencies can lead to ariboflavinosis, which is a disorder that leads to a lower level of a protein important in energy metabolism. Symptoms include inflammation of the throat and mouth, development of a magenta tongue, decreased red blood cell number, and various dermatological disorders and rashes.
- **Vitamin B3 (niacin):** Deficiencies of this vitamin are generally associated with tryptophan deficiencies and can lead to Pellagra which has symptoms of photosensitivity, increased aggression, skin lesions, weakness, confusion, dementia and diarrhea.
- **Vitamin B5 (pantothenic acid):** Deficiencies of this vitamin have been associated with increased acne. Vitamin B5 deficiencies can also lead to the development of paresthesia, a numbness of the skin.

Vitamins B6, B7, B9, B12

Vitamin B6, B7, B9, and B12 deficiencies are described below:

- **Vitamin B6 (pyridoxine)**: Deficiency can lead to peripheral neuropathy, anemia, and in severe cases, seizures.
- **Vitamin B7 (biotin)**: Deficiency in children can lead to stunted growth and various neurological problems.
- **Vitamin B9 (folic acid)**: Deficiency can lead to an up regulation of homocysteine. Folic acid deficiencies in pregnancy can lead to severe birth defects. There is evidence that folic acid can be beneficial against cancer as well. Folic acid deficiency can also lead to decreased RNA and DNA synthesis in red blood cells leading to increased red blood cell size and increased anemia.
- **Vitamin B12 (cobalamin)**: Deficiency can lead to pernicious anemia, an anemia strictly associated with B12 vitamin. It can also lead to decreased cognition and memory lapse as well as decreased RNA and DNA synthesis in red blood cells, leading to increased red blood cell size and increased anemia.

Hypokalemia and Hyperkalemia

Hypokalemia occurs in response to low potassium levels, generally levels **less than 3.5 mEq/L.** Hypokalemia can be caused by decreased intake of potassium due to poor diet. It can also be caused by increased loss of potassium due to drugs such as corticosteroids, diuretics, amphotericin B, and laxative abuse. Symptoms include cardiovascular (hypotension, differences in EKG), neuromuscular (cramps, weakness, lack of reflexes), and renal (unable to excrete concentrated urine, excess water loss) changes. **Hyperkalemia** is due to high potassium levels, generally levels **greater than 5.5 mEq/L.** Hyperkalemia can occur due to decreased effectiveness of potassium excretion, which can be due to renal dysfunction or certain drugs such as spironolactone. Hyperkalemia can also be caused by excessive cellular breakdown, excessive intake due to supplements or IV fluids, and metabolic acidosis. Symptoms include bradycardia and hypotension.

Hyponatremia and Hypernatremia

Hyponatremia occurs when sodium levels fall below normal physiological levels, **less than 125 mEq/L.** Hyponatremia occurs in response to both increased fluid levels and dilution of fluids in response to various disease states including cirrhosis of the liver, congestive heart failure, renal failure and syndrome of inappropriate ADH. It can also be caused by excessive sodium depletion due to kidney failure, sodium wasting, and severe decrease of sodium intake from the diet. Symptoms include edema, cramps, confusion, dizziness, seizures and comas. **Hypernatremia,** however, occurs when sodium levels are excessive, **greater than 150 mEq/L.** This is often caused by dehydration, which can be due to not drinking enough water. Several drugs known as diuretics can increase sodium levels in the body. Excessive intake of sodium through diet, drugs and IV fluids can also result in hypernatremia. Symptoms include thirst, overactive reflexes, seizures, and even death.

Hypercholesteremia

Hypercholesteremia is a symptom of a more serious underlying disorder and occurs due to increased levels of cholesterol in the blood. It is closely related to hyperlipidemia, which is the increased level of lipids in the blood. Increased cholesterol is associated with atherosclerotic plaques, which can impede blood flow leading to hypertension and have important deleterious effects leading to heart disease. Total cholesterol levels below or equal to 200 mg per dL of blood are considered optimal. 200–239 mg/dL of cholesterol are considered marginally high, while cholesterol levels greater than 239 are considered overtly high. The presence of lipoproteins such as LDL and HDL is associated with cholesterol levels and are also measured as cholesterol levels. LDL in a healthy individual should remain lower than 100 mg/dL. LDL levels of 100–189 mg/dL are considered moderately elevated to high level. LDL over 189 is considered severely high. HDL level of 40–60 mg/dL is considered optimal, less than 40 is considered low, while greater than 60 is considered high.

Hypertriglyceridemia

Hypertriglyceridemia occurs when blood level of triglycerides are increased. Triglycerides are usually the most abundant of the lipids that are found in the body and at reasonable levels are a good source of energy, but can lead to severe health problems if levels are increased including heart disease and diabetes. Triglycerides in a healthy individual with low risk of developing heart disease and other disorders should be lower than 150 mg/dL in the blood. Triglyceride levels of 150–200 mg/dL are considered slightly to intermediately high with increased risk of developing heart disease. Levels of 200–499 mg/dL are considered high, while levels greater than 499 mg/dL are considered severely high, with a very high risk of developing heart disease.

Effects of Teratogenic Drugs on Development of Fetus

During the first two weeks of gestation, the fertilized zygote divides, and implementation occurs in the uterus. During these approximately first two weeks, the basic developmental properties that give rise to the more complex organ development are formed. Teratogenic drugs and other insults to the fetus at this point rarely lead to developmental disorders, however, they can lead to spontaneous abortion, sometimes before the mother even realizes she is pregnant. During the next six-seven weeks, the heart, limbs and ears develop. Eyes develop from four to thirty-eight weeks, while the central nervous systems and peripheral nervous systems develop from three to thirty-eight weeks. Teratogenic drugs, radiation, infectious agents and other fetal damaging agents can potentially harm fetal development throughout the pregnancy.

Irritable Bowel Syndrome

Irritable bowel syndrome (IBS) can present clinically with abdominal pain, diarrhea and/or constipation, heartburn, nausea, cramps, increased urination, and decreased sexual desire. IBS is one of the most common diseases of the digestive system. IBS is also more common in women. First line therapy in patients with a mild case of IBS includes antimuscarinic and anticholinergic drugs such as dicyclomine and hyoscyamine. Laxatives can help with constipation, but does not affect other IBS symptoms. Loperamide is a drug that is used to treat against diarrhea, but does not affect other IBS symptoms. Other drugs used to treat this disorder include selective serotonin reuptake inhibitors and tricyclic antidepressants. Tegaserod is a serotonin agonist which can relieve various IBS symptoms, including bloating and pain, and helps in constipation IBS. Alosetron was a serotonin antagonist that was used to treat IBS with diarrhea, but was pulled from the market due to a possible connection to increased cardiac distress. Tricyclic antidepressants and antimuscarinic and anticholinergic drugs can lead to depression of the central nervous system, constipation, decreased sweating, urine retention and decreased urination. Tegaserod can lead to increased nausea, headache, and abdominal pain. Laxatives can lead to cramping and if overused can lead to the loss of important bacterial colonies from the gut, as well as damage to the GI tract.

Peptic Ulcer Disease

Peptic ulcers are a general classification of lesions of the GI tract usually due to excessive acid or other digestive enzymes. Ulcers can also be caused by infections from the Helicobacter pylori, gram-negative bacteria, NSAIDs and stress. Clinically, symptoms often occur after eating and pain, and are relieved by antacids or other drugs such as PPIs. Pain can exist from hours to months, depending on how serious and large the ulcer is. Pain can be relatively acute and can lead to chronic pain. Treatment includes relieving symptoms and underlying causes/infections. For helicobacter pylori infections, antibiotic drug regimens can be used. For NSAID induced peptic ulcers, removal of NSAID use will often help. Antacids can also be used; other drugs such as proton pump inhibitors (PPI) and H2-receptor blocker are drugs that can be used to inhibit release of gastric juices, allowing ulcers to heal. Drug regimens of these drugs can often be chronic.

Review Video: Peptic Ulcers
Visit mometrix.com/academy and enter code: 184332

Ulcerative Colitis

Ulcerative colitis (UC) is a type of inflammatory bowel disease. It affects the colon and rectum. The most common clinical symptom of ulcerative colitis that generally appears first includes bloody diarrhea, as well as a painful and frequent need to defecate. UC is often caused by inflammation and ulcers. UC severity (mild, moderate, severe and fulminate) are diagnosed by endoscopy, tissue biopsy, and bacterial studies of feces. UC is considered mild if defecation occurs less than four times a day, marred with or without blood and with a normal erythrocyte sedimentation rate. Moderate UC has more than four defecations a day with signs of toxicity (little bleeding, low levels of infection, etc.) Patients with severe UC suffer from six or more defecations with noticeable systemic symptoms including fever, anemia, infection, etc. Fulminate UC occurs if there are ten or more defecations a day with significant levels of systemic symptoms, including abdominal distention, continuous bleeding and may need numerous blood transfusions. Treatment can include drugs as well as surgery.

Crohn's Disease

Crohn's disease (CD) is a type of irritable bowel disease which leads to inflammation of the GI tract which can affect any part of the GI tract, from the mouth to the anus. CD is chronic, although symptoms may go into remission for periods of time. Certain factors that might lead to CD may be bacterial infection or overeating; however, the exact cause is not entirely understood. Symptoms of CD can include chronic diarrhea, frequent bouts of diarrhea at night, and increased levels of abdominal pain. CD is marred by lesions of the GI tract. Other symptoms can include fever, excessive bleeding from the rectum, and may lead to weight loss as well as excessive fatigue. CD also can also have non-GI related symptoms including the development of arthritis, formation of painful nodules on the limbs, fatty liver, hepatitis, and gallstones. Treatment can include drugs as well as surgery.

Risk Factors Associated with Acute Pancreatitis

There are many risk factors associated with **acute pancreatitis** such as alcohol consumption, certain insect venoms and insecticides. Infectious diseases, vascular problems including atherosclerosis and vasculitis, hypertriglyceridemia, hypercalcemia, gallstone disease, cystic fibrosis, inflammatory bowel disease, and peptic ulcer disease also are associated with acute pancreatitis. Also, many medications have been associated with acute pancreatitis, including 5-aminosalicyclic acid, asparaginase, azathioprine, didanosine, furosemide, mercaptopurine, methyldopa, metronidazole, pentamidine, sulfonamides, sulindac, tetracyclines, thiazides, and valproic acid.

Chronic Pancreatitis

Chronic pancreatitis (CP) is usually caused by structural damage to the pancreas and is often associated with chronic inflammation. The patient may show symptoms of malnutrition. Additionally, CP is often associated with liver disease brought on by chronic alcoholism. Symptoms of pancreatitis include deep dull pain in the abdomen with nausea and vomiting. CP is often associated with excessive weight loss and excessive loss of fat and protein through the feces (steatorrhea and azotorrhea respectively). The use of analgesics such as aspirin, acetaminophen, and ibuprofen are used as treatment for the pain while anti-inflammatory drugs such as NSAIDS and COX-2 are used for the inflammation of the pancreas. Non-pharmacological treatment includes stopping alcohol ingestion and the introduction of a fat reduced diet.

Congestive Heart Failure

Congestive heart failure (CHF) occurs when structural or functional damage occurs to the heart that leads to a significant decrease in heart function. This is often due to a lower force of the heart beat as well as incomplete filling of the heart with blood before each contraction, thus lowering the effectiveness of blood pumped to the body. Failure of the left side of the heart can lead to shortness of breath, cough, confusion, excessive sweating, and excessive chilliness of the limbs. Failure of the right side of the heart can lead to excessive edema in the limbs and the abdominal cavity, nightly bouts of urination, excessive nosebleeds, and enlarged liver. Drugs that are used to treat CHF include digoxin, ACE inhibitors, diuretics, β-blockers, and vasodilators.

New York Heart Association Functional Guidelines of Heart Failure

The New York Heart Association functional guidelines of heart failure are as follows:

- **Functional Class I**: Patients with heart disease that does not hinder activity at all.
- **Functional Class II**: Patients with heart disease that shows minor hindrance of physical activity, increased tiredness, increased odd heart rate, fluttering of the heart, and increased chances of chest pain and angina.

- **Functional Class III**: Patients with moderate to severe hindrance of physical activity of patients, there are no obvious symptoms of heart disease except at rest.
- **Functional Class IV**: Patients with heart disease/heart failure symptoms are present at all times, including at rest.

Heart Failure Management Guidelines

The heart failure management guidelines from the American College of Cardiology/American Heart Association are listed below:

- **Stage A**: There are no symptoms or presence of heart failure, however, patients have a high risk of contracting disease (i.e. genetics, obesity, and hypertension)
- **Stage B**: Patients develop physical signs/damage to the heart as an indicator of heart failure, but do not show other symptoms of the disease
- **Stage C**: Patients that have current symptoms of heart disease or past symptoms with underlying structural damage to the heart.
- **Stage D**: Patients with severe damage to the heart and severe symptoms of heart disease.

Osteoarthritis

Osteoarthritis is a disease that leads to the degenerative breakdown of the cartilage in joints. Cartilage protects our joints by acting as a cushion and can protect the wearing of our bones. When the cartilage degrades, this protection of the joints is lost, leading to stiffness and pain. Osteoarthritis is known to affect the hips, hands, feet, knees and spine. Osteoarthritis is often a component of age; the joints become increasingly inflamed which can lead to pain and swelling. In advanced cases, total loss of cartilage can occur, severely limiting mobility of the patient. Other causes of osteoarthritis include obesity, surgery on the joints, diabetes, and gout. Treatment exists for limiting pain, with such medicines as acetaminophen and aspirin. Weight loss can limit progression,

Gout

Gout is a disease that occurs in response to high levels of uric acid that deposit in the joints, leading to pain and inflammation. Gout is caused by hyperuricemia. The incidence of gout has been reported for millennia and is known to occur in 1% of the population. Symptoms generally begin with pain in the joints of the feet. During an arthritis attack the patient can experience a fever, and the affected area can be very inflamed and tender to the touch. Treatment against a gouty arthritis attack including colchicine. Colchicine acts as an anti-inflammatory agent and acts by inhibiting leukocyte phagocytosis of uric acid crystals. Diarrhea and cramping can occur, and patients should be counseled to stop taking this drug once it occurs. This drug can also cause bone marrow depression. Indomethacin and corticosteroids can also be used to treat acute gouty arthritis.

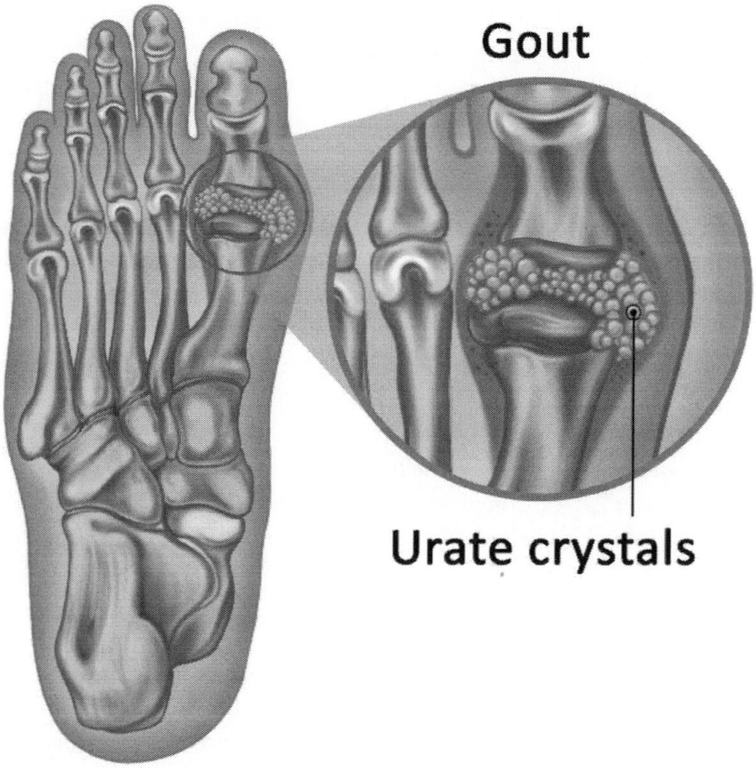

RHEUMATOID ARTHRITIS

Rheumatoid arthritis (RA) is an autoimmune disease that causes the immune system to attack the joints. As the disease progresses, the pain and loss of mobility can be severe, and other tissues including the heart, lungs and muscles may be affected. Rheumatoid arthritis has an incidence of 1% and usually affects women more than men between the ages of 30 and 60. Clinical symptoms can progress unpredictably. Ten to twenty percent of patients with this disease have a short disease, with a long remission; seventy to eighty percent have a moderate form of the disease with continual cyclical outbreaks. Ten to twenty percent; the disease will continue to progress into a rather destructive disease. Patients meet at least four criteria: morning stiffness that lasts at least 1 hour, swelling of three or more areas of soft tissue around the joints with systemic arthritis, positive rheumatoid factors which are antibodies that collect in joints, erosion of bones around joints, or nodules that form over points of arthritic joints but beneath the skin.

GENERALIZED SEIZURES

Generalized seizures occur on both sides of the brain and include:

- **Absence seizures** are subtle seizures that last only a few seconds, include a loss of awareness, but usually not complete unconsciousness. People with this disorder will often stare blankly, completely unaware of their surroundings. Often occurring in children, these seizures are hard to diagnose, and will often go unnoticed for years.
- **Atonic seizures** lead to a complete loss of muscle strength or tone, often causing the victim to collapse suddenly. There is little warning, and protective helmets and clothing are often worn in case the patient falls.
- **Myoclonic seizures** are rapid whole-body muscle contractions. Contractions are brief and usually occur on both sides of the body at the same time (e.g., arms or legs).

- **Tonic clonic seizures**, also known as grand mal seizures, are the most common seizure type. Often affecting the entire body, first the body stiffens (tonic) and becomes very rigid, next severe muscle contraction and jerking occurs (clonic). Loss of respiratory function can also occur.

Partial Seizures

Partial seizures are the most common seizures attributed to patients suffering from epilepsy. Partial seizures are generally caused by a disturbance in the electrical activity of a specific region in the brain. There are two types of partial seizures: simple partial seizures and complex partial seizures. During simple partial seizures, patients do not lose consciousness; the seizure can originate at one point in the body, leading to rapid contraction of muscles but can eventually spread to be a more general-like seizure. These seizures are often attributed to unusual sensations of taste, touch, smell, hearing and sight. They can also bring about odd exaggerated emotional states including fear, rage, anger and even joy. A person having complex seizures may appear conscious, however, they do not remember anything that has occurred during the seizure, what was said, or what was felt. Complex partial seizures largely affect the temporal lobe of the brain and affect more of the brain function than simple partial seizures.

Typical Migraine Headaches

Migraines are a certain type of headache that is often associated with nausea, light sensitivity, audio sensitivity and sensitivity to smells. Migraines are generally chronic and can last from a few hours to a couple of days. Pain caused by migraines can differ from patient to patient and is often an intense throbbing. Migraines can be associated with auras, which are neurological changes that occur about thirty minutes before the onset of the headache. These auras are often visual changes such as hallucinations, blurry images, vision loss, lights, etc. Some patients have migraines that are not associated with auras. Migraine triggers are often patient specific, but can include allergies, food, too much or too little sleep and hormonal changes. It is suggested that the pain of a migraine headache is due to excessive vasodilation in the blood vessels of the brain. This increased pressure in the head, leads to this pain, although the exact causes of a migraine are not entirely understood.

Atypical Migraine Headaches

Besides the normal migraines with or without an aura, **other types of migraines** also exist such as abdominal migraine, basilar type migraine, familial hemiplegic migraine and acephalgic migraine. Abdominal migraines often affect children and are associated with nausea, abdominal pain, as well as flushing of the skin or draining of the skin, loss of appetite and can last up to 72 hours. Treatment can include anti-nausea medicine (promethazine), triptans (anti-migraine), NSAIDs, and other anti-migraine medicine. Basilar artery migraines occur in response to a malfunction within the brainstem, due to errors in vasodilation of the basilar artery, which can lead to headache, dizziness and loss of muscle coordination. Treatment can include vasoconstrictors and triptans. Acephalgic (headache-free) migraines occur when a patient experiences normal migraine symptoms, including photosensitivity, audiosensitivity, nausea, and auras, but they do not experience a headache. These will often gradually become a more classical migraine with a headache. Treatment can include anti-nausea medicine (promethazine), triptans (anti-migraine), NSAIDs, and other anti-migraine medicine.

Meningitis

Meningitis can be caused by numerous microbial organisms, including gram negative organisms such as E.Coli, as well as Group B streptococci such as Haemophilus influenzae, Neisseria meningitides, and Streptococcus pneumoniae and listeria monocytogenes. Meningitis occurs when the protective membranous layer surrounding the central nervous system known as the meninges becomes inflamed. A spinal tap is often performed to measure levels of white blood cells in the cerebrospinal fluid. An excess of white blood cells can indicate meningitis. Patients will often have a fever, aversion to light, nausea, diarrhea, and change in mental acuity. Initial treatment of meningitis, before actual diagnosis is known, which is known as empiric therapy differs with age. Treatment of meningitis usually consists of a regimen of cefotaxime or ceftriaxone alone or in combination with vancomycin, or a combination regimen of ampicillin with aminoglycoside or vancomycin. Generally these antibiotics do not readily get to the sight of infection, and thus the highest safe dose of the antibiotic is generally given.

Review Video: Meningitis
Visit mometrix.com/academy and enter code: 277418

Endocarditis

The most common cause of **endocarditis** is *Streptococcus* and *Staphylococcus*, which can cause infections in the protective lining of the heart. This type of infection is more common in patients already suffering from some heart damage and may have had some heart surgery in the past. Patients will be fatigued and feverish, and generally diagnosis will occur through visual inspection. Treatment can depend on the causative microbial agent that led to the infection. In streptococcus, penicillin G alone or in combination with gentamycin can be given. Additionally, ceftriaxone can also be given. In staphylococcus infections, nafcillin, oxacillin, and cefazolin can be given alone or in combination with gentamycin. In both cases of streptococcus and staphylococcus infections, vancomycin can also be given if penicillin offers potential complications.

Cystic Fibrosis

Cystic fibrosis is a heritable genetic disorder in response to a genetic mutation that leads to a mutated protein known as cystic fibrosis transmembrane regulator (CFTR), which is an important channel that is involved in the transport of water and electrolytes such as Cl-. This disease leads to excessive mucosal production which can cause severe defects in the function of various organs, including defects of the pancreas, intestine and lungs. Cystic fibrosis can also lead to cirrhosis of the liver, arthritis, anemia, and diabetes. In the lungs, excessive mucous production can lead to: increased bacterial infections, increased bacterial colonization, bronchiolitis and chronic blockage in the lungs. Cystic fibrosis cannot be cured and treatment is focused on reduction of infections and reduction of chronic symptoms with the goal of prolonging life. Treatments include pancreatic enzymes; insulin; N-Acetylcysteine, which can lower mucous levels; bronchodilators; anti-inflammatory drugs; etc.

Celiac Disease

Celiac disease is an autoimmune disorder that affects the small intestine. It occurs in people genetically disposed to the disease. Often the disease is exacerbated by the presence of gliadin, a gluten glycoprotein found in wheat. In response to the interaction of the protein tissue transglutaminase with gluten, an autoimmune reaction occurs, leading to inflammation of the small intestine. This inflammation causes a decrease in nutrient absorption. Symptoms can include weight loss, increased tiredness, excessive diarrhea and gas. In children, the disease can lead to stunted growth. Other symptoms can include abdominal pain and ulcer formations. If gone unchecked, it can also lead to malnutrition and the development of cancer. Blood tests are performed to measure levels of IgA antibodies which are common for celiac disease. One of the most common and most effective treatments is the removal of gluten from the diet. Sometimes, however, celiac disease becomes resistant to diet alone, and this is known as the refractory portion of the disease. Steroids and immunosuppressants can be used for treatment.

Sickle Cell Anemia

Sickle cell anemia is a genetic disorder in which a point mutation of hemoglobin occurs, which can lead to blood cells taking on a sickle shape. These sickle-shaped blood cells often have increased damage to the cellular membrane of the cells due to the warped shape. Life expectancy is relatively less; however patients usually live a quality life. Often patients will suffer from periodic painful sickle crisis. Sickle cell crisis is often called vaso-occlusive crisis, which occurs when sickle blood cells clump and block important blood vessels to organs, leading to possible organ damage as well as pain. A common type of vaso-occlusive crisis is known as acute chest crisis and includes chest pains, struggled breathing, and fever. Symptoms often resemble pneumonia. Treatment includes oxygen, and antibiotics as well as NSAIDS and other opioids. Other sickle cells crise include aplastic crisis (exacerbation of anemia leading to increased paleness, irregular heart rate, and tiredness) and splenic sequestration crisis (acute enlargement of the spleen, often painful).

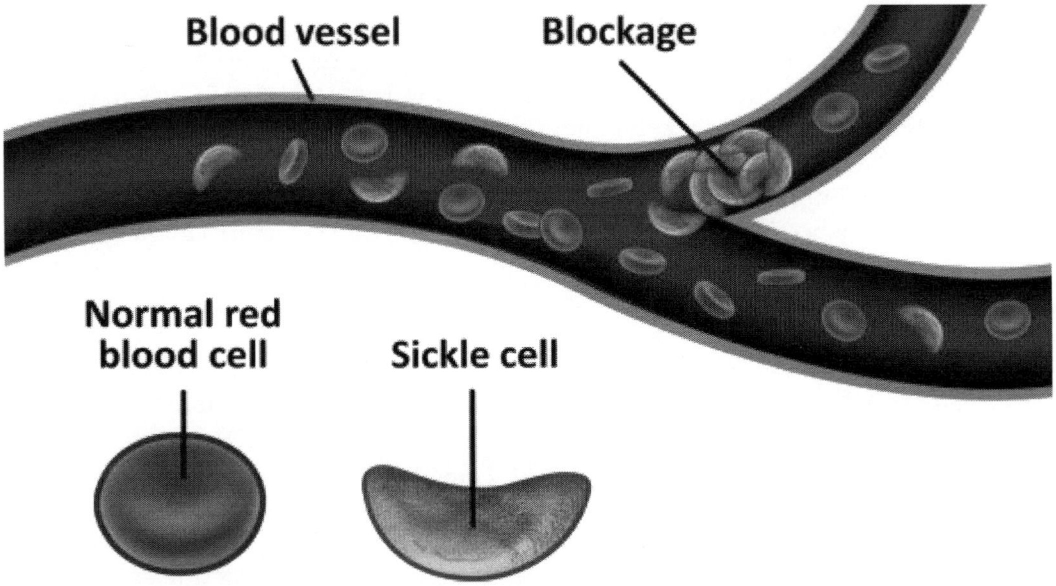

Review Video: Sickle Cell Disease
Visit mometrix.com/academy and enter code: 603869

Anemia of Chronic Disease

Anemia of chronic disease (ACD), or anemia of inflammation, is one of the most common forms of anemia which has been connected to inflammation, tissue damage, as well as infectious diseases. This anemia is characterized by shortened blood cell lifespan, decreased bone marrow response to erythropoietin, and iron sequestration. Infections that are linked with ACD include tuberculosis, HIV, bacterial endocarditis, and chronic UTIs. Chronic inflammatory diseases such as osteoarthritis, rheumatoid arthritis, gout, and lupus erythematosus are also linked to ACD. Cancer and other diseases such as alcohol induced liver disease, congestive heart failure and other heart disease can lead to ACD as well.

Symptoms Scores Related to Severity of BPH

BPH (benign prostatic hyperplasia) is a disorder of elderly men, a non-malignant growth of the prostate that can lead to discomfort, particularly during urination. According to the American Urological Association a symptom score equal or less than seven equates to mild BPH. Mild BPH is associated with a maximum rate of urination at 10 mLs per second and increased urinary retention (from 25mL up to 50mL). Additionally. BUN levels and creatinine levels are increased in the serum.

Moderate BPH has a symptom level between 8 and 19. Moderate BPH has symptoms of mild BPH with increased irritation and feelings of obstruction during urination. A BPH AUA symptom score above 20 is considered severe, which includes the above symptoms along with other problems such as urinary tract infections, kidney damage and incontinence.

Non-Prescription Drug Treatments for Common Cold

The **common cold** is often a highly contagious viral infection, leading to respiratory distress. Symptoms can include a low fever, sore throat, cough, nasal congestion, and general lethargy. Possible nonprescription drug suggestions can include decongestants (to relieve sinus pressure and mucous build-up and to make breathing easier), anti-histamines to decrease runny noses and allow for easier sleep, NSAIDs and other analgesics for pain, headaches and fever, and local numbing agents (topical anesthetics to treat the sore throat). Common decongestants include phenylephrine, pseudoephedrine; common anti-histamines can include diphenhydramine, loratadine; common analgesics include aspirin, ibuprofen, acetaminophen, local numbing agents/anesthetics include benzocaine, menthol and phenol.

Rashes Caused By Poison Ivy, Poison Oak, and Poison Sumac

Poison ivy, poison oak, and poison sumac can lead to allergic skin reactions known as rhus dermatitis. Most people are sensitive to the sap from the leaves, stems, and roots of the rhus family of plants, but like any allergy, it is acquired. Generally, the allergy occurs due to direct contact of the sap on the skin. Rashes can range from mild to severe. Rashes are usually itchy, and painful fluid filled blisters generally form on the skin. Rash may appear a few hours up to a week after exposure, and symptoms can last nearly a month. Rash can spread to other parts of the body in response to itching. These rashes are not contagious. They will clear up after a few weeks untreated if mild. Other treatments can include OTC local anesthetics, hydrocortisone products, and agents that dry oozing blisters and dry up rashes (calamine lotion, aluminum sulfate, zinc oxide, etc.) Cool compresses can also be useful.

Traveler's Diarrhea

Traveler's diarrhea is a very common occurrence when a patient travels, especially to developing nations. In fact, up to 50% of people traveling experience some type of diarrhea. The risk of traveler's diarrhea can be reduced by not drinking tap water and only eating cooked food or fruits that have been personally peeled. It is also important to remind patients to use bottled water for brushing teeth and to avoid swallowing any water in the shower. If a patient does develop traveler's diarrhea, it is usually self-limiting and can be improved by staying hydrated and by taking 4mg Loperamide. If a patient has a fever or is experiencing bloody stools, they should not take Loperamide and will most likely need antibiotic therapy. Fluoroquinolones are often used with very good success and are only needed for about 3 days.

Alopecia

Androgenic alopecia (male pattern baldness) occurs in the presence of excessive androgen, a common component of aging in males. Other types of alopecia can occur in response to chemotherapy, hereditary and other underlying diseases, but these often are untreatable. Minoxidil (Rogaine) and finasteride (Propecia) can be used to treat male pattern baldness. The mechanism of action of minoxidil is not understood; it may stimulate hair follicle cellular growth and may also increase blood flow to hair follicles encouraging growth. Minoxidil is applied in 1 ml doses, twice daily and must be applied continuously for continuous hair growth. Adverse effects include excessive hair growth all over the body, possible increased heart rate, and should not be used on a pregnant female. Finasteride was originally used to treat benign prostatic hyperplasia and prostate cancer. Finasteride inhibits 5-α-reductase by inhibiting testosterone conversion to dihydrotesterosterone. DHT is important in hair loss. Finasteride is usually taken once a day for three months to see if it works. Side effects include breast enlargement, skin rashes, erectile dysfunction, decreased sex drive and can be teratogenic.

Symbiotic Host-Parasite Relationships

The following are three types of symbiotic host-parasite relationships:

- **Mutualism**: In this case, the host parasite relationship is beneficial to both organisms. An example of this could be the many types of bacteria we have in our GI tract that aid us in digestion and breaking down some of our nutrients.
- **Commensalism**: Occurs when there may be a benefit to one of the organisms, usually the parasite, but it does not injure the host, nor does it offer any apparent help. An example of this includes insects that use larger animals not as a source for food, but as transportation. It helps the insect, but does not cause any real harm to the host animal.
- **Parasitism**: Occurs when organism thrives through the expense of another organism. An example of this could be seen with infectious microbial agents. They need other organisms to thrive, however, this leads to disease and sometimes death to the host.

Giardiasis

Giardia Lamblia is a parasitic protozoan that affects the gastrointestinal system and is the most common cause of diarrhea. *Giardia* is usually caused by ingesting water contaminated with fecal matter. The low pH of the stomach causes the release of the trophozoite, a protozoan with flagella, which can reproduce and colonize in the small intestine and can cause numerous problems of the gastrointestinal system including excessive edema, destruction of cilia, which severely decreases the absorption of nutrients, inducing severe diarrhea and dehydration. Can also lead to abdominal pain, gas, nausea, and can cause malnutrition. Diagnosed patients should be treated with metronidazole (250 mg TID for 7 days), furazolidone (100 mg QID for 7days), or paromomycin (25–30 mg a day for 7 days). Pediatric doses differ metronidazole (15 mg TID for seven days), furazolidone (6 mg/kg QID for seven days), and nitazoxanide suspension (100 -200 mg every 12 h for three days). Another pediatric drug that can be used is albendazole (400 mg daily for a week).

Scabies

Scabies occurs due to an infestation of the Sarcoptes scabiei mite, an insect that can cause severe itching of the skin. Scabies is usually transmitted from person to person, and since they can live up to 36 hours on the human host, infestation can occur by touching clothes or bed sheets that may be infested, while not actually touching a person. At the beginning mild itching is common, which quickly intensifies particularly at night. Eczema and rashes can also form. These mites usually make burrows into the skin, creating small little scratch-like marks on the skin which is often used for diagnosis. Treatment includes OTC products such as permethrin which can kill the mites. Oral medication known as ivermectin has shown to be effective in curing scabies. Diphenhydramine, an OTC antihistamine medication can ease itching.

Lice

Three species of lice can infest the human host: head (Pediculus humanus capitis), body (Pediculus humanus corporis) and pubic (Pthirus pubis). Head lice are the most common forms of infestation and are mostly found in the hair on top of the head. Head lice can be found on anyone, cleanliness does not necessarily matter. Body lice are more common in poverty-stricken nations and people. Body lice are found in clothing, but use the body as a food source. Pubic lice, also known as crab lice, are generally found in the pubic hair, which can also travel to the eyebrows and eyelashes. Pubic lice are a sexually transmitted disease. Most common symptoms are itching, possible formation of welts from the biting insects and rash formation. Treatment for lice includes OTC treatments of permethrin (a plant derivative that has several forms of chrysanthemic and pyrethic acid which is deadly to the lice). For NIX resistant lice, another OTC product known as Ovide (malathion) could be used.

Malnutrition

Malnutrition is caused by under-nutrition and obesity. Under-nutrition occurs in response to starvation or a change in metabolism of nutrients, which might be caused by injury, in which the proper dietary needs are not being met. Obesity occurs when there is too much caloric intake, which often coincides with lack of exercise. Genetic traits can also increase chances of obesity. There are three types of obesity; type I has a body mass index (BMI) greater than 30 but less than thirty-five; type II obesity are patients that have a BMI between 35 and 40, and types III, which has patients with a BMI over 40. Other types of malnutrition include marasmus, which are patients that have low levels of fat and muscle, but otherwise appear healthy. Kwashiorkor, are patients that have normal or slightly higher levels of fat and muscle, but show low immune response and low levels of important biochemical enzymes and proteins. People can also suffer a mixture of Kwashiorkor and marasmus in which fat, muscle, the immune response, and enzyme, protein and metabolic pathways are retarded.

Causes of Developmental Defects

Developmental defects can be caused by any of the following:

- **Chromosomal defects**: Occurs usually early during development, commonly an extra chromosome exists known as trisomy. Trisomy 13 has been linked to the disease holoprosencephaly, which is due to the lack of forebrain development, which can cause severe facial and brain deformities.
- **Infectious diseases**: Certain diseases can lead to various abnormal developments of the fetus. Rubella can cause Congenital Rubella syndrome (CRS) in unborn fetus. CRS can lead to abnormal heart, eye and brain development. Children are generally intellectually disabled, underweight and have smaller heads.
- **Teratogenic drugs**: Certain drugs can lead to abnormal development of the fetus.
- **Deficiencies**: Deficiencies of certain vitamins are hormones often can lead to abnormal fetal development. One example is folic acid; increased folic acid levels can decrease chances in developing neural tube defects.
- **Radiation**: Can lead to various severe developmental deformities depending on time frame of pregnancy exposure occurred and length of exposure.

Mania and Depression

Manic episodes have several characteristics which include increased hyperemotional states which can include feelings of increased euphoria and joy, rapid and quick speech, increased agitation, as well as increased energy. Often people experiencing manic episodes also suffer from mild to severe insomnia depending on the severity of the manic episode. People suffering from mania often cannot function properly in life or at work and may experience psychotic episodes. **Depression** has several symptoms that include fatigue, increased sleep as well as insomnia, altered appetite, feelings of helplessness, increased unwarranted feelings of guilt, hopelessness, and anxiety. Often depressive episodes involve suicidal thoughts. People who suffer from bipolar disorders will suffer from varying cyclical bouts of mania and depression.

Data Collection and Data Assessment

Importance of Obtaining a Full Patient History

There are several things that should be covered when obtaining a **comprehensive patient history**. Identifiers such as name, date of birth, sex, the name of their family physician, race and nationality should be recorded. When obtaining a history, it is important to be respectful and polite, if a patient is comfortable, they are more willing to provide private information. Complaints (reasons for the patients visit), how long the symptoms have progressed, current and past medical care, allergies, present drug prescriptions, as well as OTC medication that the patient may be on should also be recorded. Additionally, data from the system review (body temp, heart rate, blood pressure, etc.) should also be recorded. Having a comprehensive history can make therapy easier, with fewer possible medical errors occurring.

BMR

Basal metabolic rate (BMR) is a metabolic measurement which should occur after a restful night of sleep, twelve hours after eating, in a comfortable environment, with no physical or emotional excitement. This measurement should indicate the basal level or basal rate of heat production and respiration in an individual. Several factors can affect BMR including age, temperature, sex, overall body surface area, pregnancy, food, and various drugs such as reserpine or hormones such as thyroxine.

Basic Assessment Techniques

A pharmacist must know and utilize **basic healthcare assessment techniques**.

- **Palpation** is the measurement of swelling or injury of a particular area by touch, such as looking for swelling of the lymph nodes which often occurs during infection.
- **Percussion** is performed when part of the body is tapped with a finger and the reverberations of sound are used to determine the presence of underlying illness. An example of this is used to listen to listen for alterations in lung function, for example.
- **Auscultation** is a technique in which a stethoscope is used to listen to sound within the body, such as heart beat. This technique is also used simultaneously with an aneroid sphygmometer, which is important in measuring blood pressure. Other techniques include checking body temperature (optimal temp~98.6 F°) and reflexes. It is important to be thorough and accurate when inspecting a patient: their life may be at stake.

PQRST

PQRST is used when assessing pain of a patient:

- **P = Palliative (painkilling) factors of pain.** What can be used to relieve the patients suffering/pain? Provoking (painful) factors of pain—what can be done to make the pain worse?
- **Q = Quality of pain.** This really involves the patient's description of the pain, the general sensations that are being felt.
- **R = Radiation or location.** Where is the pain located in the body?
- **S = Severity.** How painful is it compared to other pains the patient may have felt before? Pain is very subjective. A scale ranging from 0–5 helps measure the severity of pain that a patient is suffering. 0 = no pain, 5 = severe pain.
- **T = Temporal factors.** Does time affect the pain? As time increases does pain decrease? Is this pain temporary, a sign of nerve damage (numbness)? Does the pain increase with time? Is the pain getting worse?

These are some of the questions you need to ask when assessing pain, as well as assessing the underlying causes of the pain, allowing for a better, more effective treatment.

Clinical Definitions of Pain

The six different clinical definitions of pain are described below:

- **Nociceptive pain**: Pain due to a stimulatory response of common pain receptors and pathways, e.g., slamming a finger in a door or reflex pain through the spinal cord due to touching a hot stove.
- **Somatic pain**: Pain in tissues that are of a somatic origin such as muscle and skin.
- **Superficial pain**: Local pain, which could feel like a burning sensation, a painful throbbing, could be due to sensitive skin, or a hypersensitivity to pain (hyperalgesia) for example.
- **Deep somatic pain**: A localized dull ache, a painful throbbing sensation.
- **Visceral pain**: Not localized, dull aching pain that often occurs at the onset of a disease
- **Neuropathic pain**: Pain that is related to direct damage to the nervous system. Could be due to injury of the peripheral nervous system or central nervous system.

Acute and Chronic Pain

Acute pain generally occurs due to an apparent injury; onset is rapid and can range from minor to severe, however, pain is relatively short lasting. Amount of pain is often proportional to the severity of the tissue damage. Acute pain is generally easier to treat since the tissue damage is generally more easily diagnosed than chronic pain. **Chronic pain** is generally considered pain that continues after apparent healing of damaged tissue has occurred. Chronic pain is difficult to manage, as the underlying causes of chronic pain are not fully understood. Also, chronic pain can become resistant to normal medical treatments. Chronic pain is also difficult to diagnose because there is often no obvious indication of the pain, unlike acute pain, where the tissue damage might be obvious. Doctors are a little more hesitant to treat chronic pain, due to some people attempting to get pain medications such as Vicodin to use for their drug addictions, rather than being in actual pain.

Pharmacologic Therapy Measures That May Alter Vital Signs

Some pharmacologic therapy may **alter vital signs** because of vasoconstriction, vasodilation, changes in heart rate, fluid/sodium/potassium retention, or unknown causes.

Hypotension

Diuretics (ex. furosemide, hydrochlorothiazide), beta-blockers (ex. metoprolol, propranolol), ACE inhibitors (ex. lisinopril, captopril), erectile dysfunction drugs (ex. sildenafil, tadalafil), anti-Parkinson drugs (ex. levodopa), TCAs (ex. amitriptyline, imipramine), sedatives (ex. zolpidem, eszopiclone), antipsychotics (ex. clozapine, olanzapine), and anxiolytics (ex. alprazolam, clonazepam, diazepam).

Hypertension

SNRIs (ex. sibutramine, venlafaxine), amphetamines, NSAIDs (ex. Ibuprofen), cox-2 inhibitors (ex. celecoxib), corticosteroids (ex. prednisone, fludrocortisone, hydrocortisone), caffeine, estrogens, progestin, and immunosuppressants (ex. cyclosporine, tacrolimus).

Bradycardia

Beta-blockers (ex. metoprolol, propranolol), digoxin, calcium channel blockers (ex. verapamil, diltiazem).

Tachycardia

Inhaled corticosteroids, albuterol, leukotriene modifiers, methylxanthine, azithromycin, pseudoephedrine, phenylephrine, SNRIs (ex. sibutramine, venlafaxine), OTC supplements (ex. valerian, ginseng, bitter orange).

Detection Rates of Drugs By Drug Tests

The detection rates of drugs by common drug tests are as follows:

- **Barbiturates** can be detected in urine for up to 3 days (long-acting barbiturates lasting longer), but up to 3 months in hair.
- **Phenylcyclohexylpiperidine (PCP)** can be detected in urine over 2 weeks after administration when used chronically, as well as 90 days in hair, and 24 hours in the blood.
- **Lysergic acid diethylamide (LSD)** can be detected for 24 hours in urine, 6 hours in blood and weeks to months in hair.
- **Cocaine** is detectible in the urine up to 4 days after administration, 24 hours in blood, and 90 days in hair.
- **Marijuana** is detectible up 3 days in the urine (may increase in habitual users), 2 days in blood, and 90 days in hair.
- **Phenobarbital** can be detected for 1–2 weeks in urine, 1 week in blood, and 90 days in hair.
- **Alcohol** can be detected for up to 12 hours in the urine and blood.

Liver Function Tests

Liver function tests measure levels of liver enzymes in the blood. Increased blood levels of these enzymes can be a sign of liver disease.

- **Alanine transaminase (ALT)** is synthesized specifically by liver cells, blood levels increase due to liver cell damage usually in response to inflammation, a common symptom of liver disease.
- **Aspartate transaminase AST**, less specific than ALT for liver damage, AST is a protein found in the mitochondria of liver cells as well as cardiac, kidney, and brain cells. When measured with ALT, however, a one to one ratio is often observed during liver damage.
- **Alkaline phosphatase (AP)** is elevated in many tissues and while it could be an indicator of liver disease, it is not specific. This should send a warning sign to look at the liver and other tissues for further diagnosis.
- Increased levels of albumin, bilirubin, Gamma-glutamyl transferase (GGT), and lactate dehydrogenase (LDH) can also indicate liver damage.

Glucose Tolerance Tests

Glucose tolerance tests are used to measure glucose levels to determine if a patient has diabetes (type I, type II, or gestational). After a period of fasting, the blood glucose levels are measured. Baseline fasting blood glucose levels are generally 70–105 mg/dL, after 30 minutes the level of glucose in the blood should be 110–170 mg/dL, which should increase to 120–170 mg/dL after 60 minutes. The fasting blood glucose levels after 90 minutes begins to drop to a range of 100–140 mg/dL and after 120 min, the level of fasting blood glucose should drop to a level of 70–120 mg/dL. These levels are optimal, and if there are deviations from these ranges, this could indicate the presence of diabetes or other underlying disorders.

PTT/APTT Test

The **PTT** test stands for the partial thromboplastin time test and it is also known as the activated PTT test. It is a diagnostic test to measure the length of time blood needs before it clots. This test is often performed at the same time as the PT test. The test is performed for a variety of reasons, but in particular to measure causes of excessive or unusual bleeding. The test is also performed to assess the presence of bleeding disorders such as hemophilia and can also be used to measure excessive clotting, which can be dangerous and fatal, if not caught in time. The test is performed to measure blood-clotting time before and after surgery. This test can be used to measure the effects of heparin, an anti-clotting agent that is often given to patients after surgery to lower the chances of developing dangerous blood clots. When the blood is taken, clotting is arrested with the addition of citrate. When the test is performed, an activator of clotting is added to the blood and the time it takes for clotting to occur is measured.

PT Test of Blood Coagulation, PR Ratio and INR

Prothrombin time (PT) is a test to measure clotting of the blood often in relation to warfarin therapy, vitamin K levels, and overall liver damage/disease. PT test provides two separate measurements including the prothrombin ratio (PR) and the international normalized ratio (INR). Thromboplastin (tissue factor) is added to the sample blood and control blood and the time for clotting is calculated. The PR is calculated by (PT of sample)/(PT of control). INR is calculated by multiplying PR by ISI. ISI is the international sensitivity index of the tissue factor that is provided by the manufacturer. It compares their tissue factor with the international standard for tissue factor and is usually between 1 and 1.5. Normal range of PT (time for blood to clot after tissue factor addition) is often 12–15 seconds. The normal INR ratio is about 0.8–1.2.

Calculating Measurements

BMI and Creatinine Clearance

The **body mass index** (BMI) is a measurement that uses height and weight as an indicator of obesity/malnutrition although this cannot be used alone to diagnose obesity. Tables are available to simplify calculations, but BMI can be calculated manually:

$$\text{BMI} = \frac{\text{Weight (kg)}}{\text{Height}^2\ (\text{m}^2)} = \frac{\text{Weight (lb)}}{\text{Height}^2\ (\text{in}^2)} \times 703$$

Resulting scores for adults age 20 and over are interpreted according to this chart:

$$\begin{aligned} < 18.5 &= \text{Underweight} \\ 18.5 - 24.9 &= \text{Normal weight} \\ 25.0 - 29.9 &= \text{Overweight} \\ \geq 30 &= \text{Obese} \end{aligned}$$

Creatinine is a waste product of protein metabolism and is filtered from the blood by the kidneys and excreted in the urine. The **creatinine clearance** test includes both a serum creatinine level and a 24-hour urine level. Creatinine clearance testing is indicated for symptoms associated with impaired renal function.

Creatinine Clearance (24-Hour Urine)

Normal values:

- Male 85–125 mL/min/1.73 m^2
- Female 75–115 mL/min/1.73 m^2

Evaluates the amount of blood cleared of creatinine in 1 minute. Approximates the glomerular filtration rate.

Serum Creatinine

Normal value: 0.6–1.2 mg/dL. Increases with impaired renal function, urinary tract obstruction, and nephritis. Level should remain stable with normal functioning.

Home Diagnostic Tests

Home diagnostic kits are used to determine pregnancy, ovulation, blood pressure, blood-glucose levels, and glucose urine levels. Several other diagnostic tools have become increasingly popular, easy to use, and easy to purchase. These devices can offer quick diagnostic views and can be used for many purposes such as an early warning for other possible more serious diseases. They are considered a nice alternative to visiting a doctor for simple tests, with not only lower costs, but less time is wasted waiting for the doctor. However, these home diagnostic kits can also be troublesome: they can be misinterpreted, thus causing unneeded worry, and important problems that might be present might be missed and ignored. These diagnostic kits might also be used in lieu of visiting the doctor, and while some home remedies might exist to treat whatever disease may be present, these kits should never be used as an alternative to a doctor's appointment.

Causes of False-Positive and False-Negative Results of Home Pregnancy Tests

False positives are rare but can result due to miscarriage in the prior few weeks or childbirth in the prior two months, or fertility pills such as Profasi, which can alter gonadotropin or hCG levels. **False negatives** can be caused by taking the pregnancy test too soon after the missed period0, using refrigerated urine and not rewarming it, or dysfunction of the pregnancy test.

Procedures for Point-of-Care Testing Devices

Blood glucose monitoring is done with a glucometer, which must be calibrated and tested regularly. Testing results from capillary blood tend to be lower than test results on venous blood. A drop of blood from a finger prick is placed on a test strip, which is inserted into the glucometer according to manufacturer's directions and the results read. Normal value: <100 mg/dL. Values of 100–125 indicate prediabetes. Hypoglycemia (low blood sugar/insulin reaction) is <70 mg/dL. Hyperglycemia is ≥160 mg/dL. **Hemoglobin A1c** home testing is done with a similar device using a drop of blood on a test strip. Diabetics should be tested at least every 3–6 months. Normal values: 4.0–5.5%. Values of 5.7–7.4% indicate prediabetes. Diabetics should generally maintain the A1c between 6 and 7.5. **Home urine drug screening** is a two-step procedure. First a urine sample is checked with a test strip to identify the presence of a substance of abuse. If a positive finding, then the urine sample is sent to a laboratory for further testing to identify the substance or determine if something, food or medicine, gave a false positive.

Patient Safety

Feeding Tubes

Feeding tubes are utilized for nourishment when a patient cannot eat on their own (due to a variety of physiologic and pathologic reasons) and IV fluids are considered insufficient. A feeding tube is generally placed into the stomach directly or into the jejunum directly for long-term needs, although feeding tubes can also be placed through the nose and down into the stomach for short term indications. A feeding tube may be placed in patients undergoing chemotherapy, patients who have swallowing issues (common after a stroke), patients who are intubated, or patients undergoing radiation. Feeding tubes can be dislodged if improperly secured (e.g., taping the tube to the abdomen). The tube site is also at risk for infection, and feeding tubes can lead to small cracks in the GI tract. More serious side effects can also occur such as hemorrhaging of the GI tract as well as leakage of gastric fluids into the body.

Drug Incompatibilities

Some **drugs are not compatible with feeding tubes**. A primary example is extended-release tablets, which cannot be crushed and therefore cannot be administered through a feeding tube. It was shown that phenytoin, an anti-seizure medicine, when administered through a feeding tube, will bind to the tube and be poorly absorbed. Normal therapeutic levels of this drug, when provided in a suspension through a feeding tube, result in subtherapeutic levels of the drug in the blood. Ciprofloxacin bioavailability levels were also significantly decreased when provided through the feeding tubes. It has also been reported that warfarin can also interact with enteral nutrition that is administered through the feeding tube. If given concomitantly with nutrients from a feeding tube, the anticoagulant nature of warfarin is significantly lessened.

Contraindications to Gradual Dose Reduction

According to OBRA '90, a **gradual dose reduction (GDR)** should be attempted within the first year after a geriatric patient has started a psychotropic medication unless otherwise contraindicated. A GDR should be tried, at a minimum, of twice a year in the first year and then annually, and if PRN dosing is also utilized, the patient's care plan should be reviewed if PRN dosing is used more than twice a week. There are certain exceptions to the GDR recommendation. Specifically, patients with a documented psychiatric illness who have had recurrent psychotic episodes and who have stabilized on a maintenance dose are exempt from gradual dose reductions. Additionally, patients with a documented psychiatric illness who have failed two previous gradual dose reductions within a year are also exempt from further gradual dose reductions.

Creating a Dosing Drug Regimen for Patients with Renal Insufficiency

Renal insufficiency occurs in response to kidney disease and failure, leading to lower clearance of various drugs, and thus new drug regimens must be designed for the patient. The important steps required for **creating a new drug regimen** include:

1. Obtaining a thorough patient medical history.
2. Determining creatinine clearance to estimate kidney function.
3. Reviewing present prescriptions and other medications of the patient.
4. Determining the correct dosing regimen of the prescriptions for the patient, the dosing regimen is individualized.
5. Monitoring clearance levels of the drugs during the new drug regimen as well as monitoring toxicity of the drugs.
6. Adjusting drug regimen based on findings of step 5, until optimal treatment is obtained. Kidney function changes as the disease progresses, thus new drug regimens will need to be adapted. State of drug clearance should constantly be monitored.

Basic Life Support

Basic life support consists of techniques to treat and sustain life long enough for the patient to reach the hospital. These techniques include first aid to treat bleeding, shock, as well as cardiopulmonary resuscitation (CPR). CPR can be used to rescue patients from cardiac and pulmonary arrest. CPR can be used to provide oxygen to the lungs of the unconscious patient by transferring oxygen mouth to mouth from one person to that of the lungs of the patient. Additionally, by providing firm chest compressions, the provider of CPR allows for blood to pump from the heart to other important organs. CPR is used as a way to sustain life until paramedics arrive, as well as possibly returning a functional heart respiratory rate to the patient. CPR has a high failure rate and patients that survive may have organ damage. CPR is meant for life support until further treatment can be performed, not a replacement for treatment.

Advanced Life Support

Advanced life support is performed as complementary treatment to basic life support, when basic life support is not sufficient. While anyone can provide basic life support, advanced life support is specific to trained healthcare professionals. Advanced life support involves the use of important medical devices including respiratory ventilators, electrocardiograms, and administration of important IV drugs. Other important advanced life support include administration of tracheal tubes to aid in breathing, chest tubes to drain excess fluids, repair of collapsed lungs, etc. A defibrillator is used to shock an irregular heartbeat back to a normal heart rate. Drugs that are commonly used include epinephrine and atropine, which both can cause an increase in heart rate. It is thought that chest compressions should be provided concomitantly with any provided advance life support.

Drug Interactions

Grapefruit-Drug Interactions

Grapefruit juice can affect the bioavailability of drugs by inhibiting the first pass effect of metabolism and by inhibiting the metabolism of cytochrome P450 enzymes. Adverse reactions occur with antihistamines, which can lead to cardiac arrhythmias. It is not safe to take with terfenadine or astemizole. There are no interactions with non-sedating histamines such as loratidine. Grapefruit juice can increase the bioavailability of anti-cholesterol drugs including simvastatin, lovastatin and atorvastatin. This could potentially lead to an increased risk of adverse reactions such as increased muscle pain, myopathy and rhabdomyoslysis. Grapefruit juice can also increase bioavailability of benzodiazepines such as diazepam and triazolam. Grapefruit juice can also interact with calcium channel blockers (nifedipine, amlodipine, nicardipine, diltiazem) and immunosuppressive drugs (cyclosporine). It is very important to counsel patients taking these medications to avoid grapefruit juice and grapefruit.

Interaction of Tyramine Rich Foods with Certain Drugs

Tyramine is a monoamine compound derived from the decarboxylation of tyrosine. Tyramine is high in many foods including aged fish, wine, overripe avocados, soy, and cheese. Many drugs can interact with foods that have high levels of tyramine. Tyramine interacts with monoamine oxidase inhibitors, affecting numerous drugs such, as furazolidone, linezolid (Zyvox), phenelzine (Nardil), tranylcypromine (Parnate) and procarbazine (Matulane). High levels of tyramine can interact with MAO inhibitors leading to a severe increase in blood pressure which can be potentially fatal. When a patient is taking these types of medications, foods rich in tyramine should be avoided. This is a very important counseling point.

Interaction of Dairy Products with Certain Medications

Dairy products (milk, cheese, and yogurt) can interact with many drugs. This interaction is most often due to the high level of calcium found in these products and is most common with medications such as: estramustine, fluoroquinolones, mycophenolate (MMF) and tetracyclines. Patients should be counseled to avoid dairy products one hour before and four hours after they take their medication. High levels of calcium will decrease the absorption of estramustine into the gut, which leads to lower than effective therapeutic level of the drug. High levels of calcium can lead to binding of calcium to fluoroquinolones, mycophenolate (MMF), and tetracyclines creating insoluble molecular complexes, which cannot absorb into the gut and therefore will render the drug useless.

Difficulty in Recognizing Drug Interactions

Drug interactions are dangerous and **sometimes hard to recognize** because the interactions may resemble a disease or new health problem, but may not necessarily be associated with a drug interaction. Drugs can interact with other drugs, which can lead to lower or higher bioavailability of the drugs; additionally a combination of drugs might lead to a separate dangerous side effect. Drugs can also interact with certain types of food. Food, similar to the drug interactions, can lead to changes in bioavailability and efficacy of the drugs. Drugs can also inhibit the absorption of necessary vitamins, nutrients, etc. from food. Many factors can regulate interactions, and as a pharmacist, these specific interactions must be well understood in order to properly counsel a patient on a particular prescription or prescriptions.

Cross Sensitivities for Latex Allergies and Penicillin Allergies

Cross sensitivity may occur when the protein in one substance to which a person is allergic is similar to a protein in another substance, causing an allergic response. Cross-sensitivity reactions:

- **Latex-fruit syndrome**: Latex is derived from the rubber plant, and those allergic to latex may react to a number of different fresh plant sources, including kiwi, avocado, potato, bell pepper, chestnut, and peach. The syndrome is believed related to IgE antibodies, which may cause an anaphylactic reaction.
- **Penicillin**: Between 2 and 7% of patients who are allergic to penicillin have a cross sensitivity to cephalosporins, but if the allergy is severe and the patient has an anaphylactic response to penicillin, the risk of cross-sensitivity to cephalosporins increases to 50%. Patients may also react to drugs that are different but in the same family, such as amoxicillin. A similar cross-sensitivity to imipenem (an IV beta-lactam) occurs.

Interaction Between Ethanol and Metronidazole

Metronidazole is an anti-microbial agent that is commonly prescribed for various disorders including giardia. Ethanol absolutely should not be ingested for several days after administration of Flagyl, due to a potentially severe drug interaction. Mixing metronidazole and ethanol can lead to a disulfiram-like reaction. This is caused by blocking acetylaldehyde dehydrogenase, leading to an increased level of acetylaldehyde in the blood. This increased level of acetylaldehyde can lead to signs of a hangover such as: headache, extreme nausea and vomiting, and flushing of the skin. This interaction can also occasionally lead to severe cardiac and liver toxicity. It is vital as a pharmacist to make sure that a patient taking Flagyl knows this potentially dangerous interaction no matter the age of the patient, as even a small amount of alcohol (such as that found in cough syrup or mouthwash) can cause a reaction.

Ethanol/Acetaminophen Interactions

Acetaminophen (Tylenol) is metabolized by one of two ways. The majority of acetaminophen is broken down in the liver by glucuronidation and sulfation and excreted from the body. Approximately 5% of the drug is converted by the P4502E1 cytochrome enzyme (CYP2E1) into a hepatotoxic compound known as N-acetyl-p-benzoquinoneimine (NAPQI). Under normal therapeutic doses, this toxic compound is quickly sequestered by glutathione. Heavy alcohol consumption (binge drinking, chronic alcoholism) can lead to an upregulation of the CYP2E1 enzyme. This up-regulation of CYP2E1 can lead to an increase of acetaminophen being metabolized into the cytotoxic NAPQI compound. If the level of NAPQI is too great, glutathione stores will be used up and the remaining NAPQI will not be able to be fully metabolized leading to potentially severe liver damage. The damage to the liver can be acute as well as chronic. An alcoholic should not consume more than 2 grams of acetaminophen a day.

Drugs That Should Not Be Crushed

There are many drugs that **should not be crushed**. While it is not feasible to memorize the complete list of these drugs, it is important to be aware of the considerations for these drugs. As a pharmacist it would be best to read all package inserts, and use common sense (e.g., if a drug is extended release, it should not be crushed, or it can lead to a possible overdose) when counseling a patient. Additionally, it is ideal to have a complete list of drugs that shouldn't be crushed available for reference.

Disease States Induced By Specific Drugs

Several disease states can be induced by specific drug use:

- **Pancreatitis**: Occurs when the pancreas becomes inflamed. Can be fatal if left untreated. Can be induced by excessive imbibing of alcohol. Can also be induced by the use of estrogens, angiotensin-converting enzyme (ACE) inhibitors (in rare instances), statins, cancer chemotherapy drugs and various other drugs including valproic acid, azathioprine, didanosine, and thiazides.
- **Nephrotoxicity**: A general term for kidney toxicity. It can be induced by NSAIDs, cisplatin, and aminoglycosides.
- **Pulmonary disease**: Pulmonary fibrosis can be induced by amiodarone and bleomycin. This occurs when scars form on the alveoli or interstitium of the lungs and the ability to transfer oxygen into the blood is damaged. Beta-blockers can lead to constriction of the bronchiole tubes. This can lead to worsening bronchospasm in patients with preexisting asthma.
- **Orthostatic hypotension**: Can be induced by numerous drugs, including α blockers, beta-blockers, ACE inhibitors, antidepressants, nitrates, and phosphodiesterase inhibitors. Orthostatic hypotension is when the blood pressure drops as the person stands up leading to severe dizziness and fainting.

Drugs Associated with Megaloblastic Anemia

Megaloblastic anemia is also known as B12-deficiency anemia. It often occurs in response to a decreased level of vitamin B12, leading to decreased nucleic acid synthesis, which can decrease DNA synthesis of red blood cell (RBC) precursors known as megaloblasts. This in turn leads to stunted RBC maturation, thus causing anemia. This anemia can often be treated with introduction of B12 by diet or dietary supplements. Several drugs have been associated with the development of megaloblastic anemia such as asazathioprine, chloramphenicol, colchicine, cyclophoshamide, cytarabine, 5-fluorodeoxyuridine, 5-fluoracil, hydroxyurea, 6-mercaptopurine, methotrexate, oral contraceptive pills, p-aminosalicylate, phenobarbital, phenytoin, primidone, pyrimethamine, sulfasalazine, tetracycline, and vinblastine.

Drugs That Can Induce Aplastic Anemia

Several drugs have been linked to inducing **aplastic anemia**. Drugs that are thought to show a strong likelihood of inducing aplastic anemia include: acetazolamide, captopril, chloramphenicol, chloroquine, chlorothiazide, chlorpromazine, dapsone, felbamate, lisinopril, lithium, pentoxifylline, quinidine, sulindac, and ticlopidine. Other drugs that seem to have some connection to aplastic anemia, although they have not been studied as extensively, include carbamazepine, diclofenac, furosemide, indomethacin, methimazole, phenobarbital, phenothiazines, phenytoin, propylthiouracil, and sulfonamides. Patients on these drugs should be monitored for signs of aplastic anemia.

Pharmacist's Role in Monitoring Drug Therapy

The pharmacist's role in **monitoring drug therapy** includes:

- **Misuse**: Note any unusual patterns of drug purchases, such as large amount of OTC cough medicines or herbal medications. Other concerns may be when patients attempt to self-medicate by refilling out-of-date prescriptions or refill prescriptions belonging to another person.
- **Abuse**: Note patients who try to fill prescriptions ahead of time or report "losing" drugs, especially controlled substances. Other indications may be changes in appearance or behavior that may indicate addictive behavior. Additionally, if prescriptions for controlled substances or other drugs that may be substituted, such as gabapentin, increase markedly from one or more physicians, this may be cause for concern. Check any state monitoring system for controlled substances for all controlled substances. Verify authenticity of prescriptions.
- **Non-adherence**: Note patients who refill prescriptions too infrequently or who ask for changes in the number of units (pills, capsules) or dosage.

Disease Prevention

Pharmacist Shortage in the United States

One big issue in the field of pharmacy is the **lack of pharmacists**. The population of the United States is expanding at an incredible degree, and more and more drugs are being prescribed to this ever-growing population every day. It is becoming extremely difficult for States to fill the need for pharmacists to match coming years will only increase marginally in relationship to the amount of prescriptions being filled. The need for pharmacists is demanding, however, to increase the number of pharmacists to match the need can lead to several problems including a greater chance of licensed pharmacists being under-qualified for the position they hold, allowing for a greater chance for medical error. Additionally, by increasing the number of pharmacists, the salary for pharmacists will begin to decline, which could have an effect on the amount of people wanting to take this job, because the salary would not match what is required from the pharmacists, thus creating a catch-22 situation.

Need for Pharmacists to Become More Specialized

As of now, pharmacists take care of a lot of different healthcare aspects when dealing with diseases and patients, however, as the needs of the population increase and healthcare needs increase, the expectations for pharmacists will also need to increase. In the future, to maintain a successful healthcare system, with increased patient care and decreased medical error, pharmacists will need to become increasingly focused, maintaining care for certain disease states, certain patient subsets, and certain types of drug regimens, much more so than is done today. This will keep the workload for the pharmacist to a feasible level and allow for better patient care with longer time with each patient, which will increase health and safety of a certain drug therapy.

Pharmacist's Role in Patient Disease Diagnosis

As a pharmacist, it is very likely that you will field many questions related to not only medications, but also to various diseases. Pharmacists will often recommend over-the-counter (OTC) medications for common ailments such as colds and coughs. It is vital to have a great understanding of all OTC medications. It is also vital to know proper dosing of all cold OTC medications for children. While OTC medications may be suggested for common ailments, the pharmacist is not legally licensed to make diagnostic decisions about a patient. If the pharmacist is ever concerned that a patient needs to be seen by a doctor for further tests, he or she should immediately counsel the patient to see a physician as soon as possible. If concerned that the patient needs immediate attention, dial 911.

Important Emerging Roles and Activities of Pharmacists

Pharmacists have had **ever-expanding important roles** in healthcare. These include:

- Maintaining a leadership position in medicine safety and efficiency in drug distribution.
- Increasing roles in direct patient care as well as improving patient care.
- Keeping up to date information of drug evidence-based guidelines to improve safety and efficacy of therapies.
- Improving the balance between patients, insurance companies and physicians; lowering costs; and improving therapy of patients.
- Taking more proactive approaches in triaging a patient to a physician or hospital.
- Managing and counseling patients on important laboratory tests.

Alternative Medicine

Alternative medicine is described as any therapy that is not considered a valid medical therapy according to the American Medical association. Although in more recent times alternative medicine is being used more frequently with traditional western medicine. Chiropractic medicine, by adjusting bones and the spine, is thought to improve not only aches and pains but also improve overall health. Prayer, also known as faith healing, surrounds the idea that religion, faith, and spirituality will help in the treatment of a disease. Acupuncture uses needles in specific pressure points in the body, thought to treat various disorders. Other alternative medicines include reiki, homeopathy, biofeedback, and other non-western medicines (medicine from Asia, Africa, and indigenous peoples).

Nonpharmacologic Therapies for Hypertension, Asthma, UTI, and diabetes

Hypertension	Reduce intake of sodium, utilize the DASH eating plan, exercise regularly, lose weight if overweight, reduce stress, practice meditation and/or relaxation exercises, and limit alcohol consumption.
Asthma	Identify and avoid triggers, stop smoking and avoid environmental smoke, exercise to tolerance regularly, reduce dust and mite exposure (clean, furniture covers), reduce mold exposure, reduce pollen exposure (keep windows closed, using air conditions and air purifiers), avoid scented products and aerosols, and stay indoors if air quality is poor.
Urinary tract infections	Maintain adequate fluid intake, avoid dehydration, and utilize appropriate perineal hygiene to avoid urethral contamination.
Diabetes	Lose weight if overweight, practice daily foot care, utilize a diabetic (low carbohydrate) diet, exercise regularly, and avoid alcohol consumption.

Nonpharmacological Treatments for Acne Vulgaris, Psoriasis, and Atopic Dermatitis

Acne vulgaris is the most common form of acne, localized inflammation on the face. Washing and scrubbing your face daily may be effective against acne, by drying and removing excess oil, dirt and bacteria. A generous washing regimen can lessen the acne impact. **Psoriasis** a common disorder leading to the reoccurrence of inflamed thickened plaques on the skin. Psoriasis has a strong genetic factor. UV light with wavelength of 310–315 nm and emollients such as lotions and creams to keep the skin hydrated can reduce the risk of a psoriasis outbreak. **Atopic dermatitis (AD)** is an itchy inflammatory disorder that is often triggered by allergens such as dust, food products, cleaning products, etc. Non-pharmacological treatment includes reduced exposure to allergen trigger of AD and moisturizing skin during AD. Diligent washing and moisturizing of the can also be used as preventative measures against AD.

Non-Pharmacological Treatment for Osteoarthritis

There are many ways a patient **can treat osteoarthritis without using drugs.** The effectiveness for the treatment will be dependent on a case by case basis, however, drugs may be the best treatment for a certain individual. Diet and exercise are an important means to treat osteoarthritis. Obesity can lead to excessive wear and tear of the joints, leading to increased pain in people suffering from osteoarthritis. Losing weight and remaining active can greatly help relieve joint pain and increase mobility. Physical therapy is also an important treatment, in which stretching and joint specific exercises can increase mobility and relieve pain of the infected joints.

Non-Drug Related Pain Management

The use of drugs in pain management is important, however, there are many **non-pharmacological methods to regulate pain** as well. These can include the use of heating pads or ice packs to relieve pain and inflammation at a site of injury. Physical therapy is also important in dealing with pain and in the healing process. Other alternative therapies which have shown benefit in the regulation of pain can include meditation, massage, and acupuncture. Alone or in combination with drugs, these alternative pain management techniques can provide a great deal of benefit to patients.

HIV Antiretroviral Therapy for Pregnant Women

A woman who has **HIV and becomes pregnant** has a 15–45% chance of passing the HIV infection to the infant. However, with appropriate management, this transmission rate can decrease to <1%. Antiretroviral therapy should be offered if the patient is not already taking any antiretroviral therapy. Ideally, two NRTIs (tenofovir with emtricitabine [or lamivudine] along with an integrase inhibitor [dolutegravir]) should be taken during the pregnancy. Pregnant women should receive continuous IV infusion of zidovudine (AZT) during labor. It is also recommended that the baby receive AZT therapy for 2–6 weeks after birth.

HIV Post-Exposure Prophylaxis

Whenever there is an exposure event, it is always important to practice **universal precautions**. In general, needle sticks make up the largest portion of infectious exposure. If you are involved in an infectious exposure, always follow the post-exposure prophylaxis protocol at your healthcare institution. Post-exposure HIV prophylaxis significantly reduces the already very slim chance of HIV infection from a needle stick. Typically HIV post-exposure prophylaxis involves two NRTIs and one other medication taken for four weeks. Follow-up HIV testing is performed several times over the next year.

Birth Control

The following are five common forms of birth control:

- **Condoms**: Made of latex, fit snugly over the penis. A condom acts as a barrier to the sperm, which collects in a reservoir at the condom tip. Condoms block pregnancy by 88% and have variable effectiveness in preventing STDs based on the infectious agent. They are easy to use, cheap, and relatively effective; however, allergies can develop against latex.
- **Diaphragm**: Latex or silicone barrier placed in the vagina, blocking sperm from reaching the cervix, inhibiting pregnancy. Diaphragms are expensive and must be fitted. When used with spermicide, they have approximately an 83% success rate in blocking pregnancy if used correctly. They provide little protection against STDs, are uncomfortable, and can increase chances of UTI.
- **Coitus interruptus**: The withdrawal method, in which the penis is removed before climaxing. This method has a high pregnancy failure rate and does not protect against STDs.
- **IUD**: Highly effective birth control device that is placed in the uterus and causes the release of leukocytes and other components that are deadly to sperm. It is not effective against STDs.
- **Oral contraceptives pills**: Using hormones, regulates menstruation and ovulation, blocks pregnancy by inhibiting follicle formation and ovulation, thickens cervical mucus, and thins the endometrium. They provide no protection against STDs, and risks of using oral contraceptives include migraines, hypertension, and strokes. Benefits include decreased risk for ovarian cancer, endometrial cancer, and acne.

IMMUNIZATIONS

An increase in life expectancy is directly associated with decreases in the death rates of children, and the one factor that has most increased survival rates of children is **immunizations**. In order to develop herd immunity (protection of a community based on a high percentage of people being immune) in most cases about 80% to 95% of the population must have immunity, depending upon the contagion of the disease. Measles, which is spread through airborne contact, for example, is more contagious than polio, which is usually spread by the fecal-oral route. Immunity may be achieved by exposure, such as having measles with its inherent risks, or by immunization, which protects against having the disease. Some diseases that were thought to be essentially eradicated, such as smallpox and polio, may reemerge if herd immunity drops. Recent increasing outbreaks of chickenpox and measles are the result of people choosing not to immunize their children often out of unfounded fears of a link between immunizations and autism.

PEDIATRIC IMMUNIZATIONS

Immunization	Schedule
Hepatitis B	3-dose series: #1 at birth (within 12–24 hours), #2 at 1–2 months, and #3 at 6–18 months.
Diphtheria, tetanus, acellular pertussis (DTaP)	<7 years, 5-dose series: #1 at 2 months, #2 at 4 months, #3 at 6 months, #4 at 15–18 months, and #5 at 4–6 years.
Tetanus, diphtheria, acellular pertussis (TdaP)	(If have not received DTaP at ≥7 years) 1 dose at 11–12 years old followed by boosters every 10 years
Rotavirus	Rotarix at 2 months and 4 months OR RotaTeq at 2 months, 4 months, and 6 months.
Haemophilus influenzae type b (Hib)	ActHib at 2 months, 4 months, 6 months and booster at 12–15 months OR PedvaxHIB at 2 months, 4 months and booster at 12–15 months.
Varicella	2-dose series: #1 at 12–15 months, #2 at 4–6 years.
Measles, mumps, rubella (MMR)	2-dose series: #1 at 12–15 months, #2 at 4–6 years.
Pneumococcal conjugate (PCV15 or PCV20)	4-dose series: 2 months, 4 months, 6 months and booster at 12–15 months.
Pneumococcal polysaccharide (PPSV23)	1 dose ≥8 weeks after PCV13 for those at high risk
Human papillomavirus (HPV)	2-dose series for boys and girls at age 11–12 (may start as young as 9) on 6- to 12-month schedule. When started at age 15 or older, a 3-dose series is recommended
Hepatitis A (HepA)	2-dose series: #1 at 12 months, #2 at 6–18 months later.
Inactivated polio (IPV)	4-dose series: 2 months, 4 months, 6–18 months, and 4–6 years.
Influenza	Yearly for children 6 months and older.
Meningococcal conjugate quadrivalent (MenACWY)	2-dose series: #1 at 11–12 years, #2 at 16 years
Meningococcal serogroup B (MenB)	Administered after shared discussion with family; 2 doses 6 months apart for teens 16–18 or ≥10 years with risk factors.

Adult/Geriatric Immunizations

Immunization	Schedule
Influenza	Yearly for all adults
TdaP or Td	1 dose if did not receive DTaP as a child AND booster every 10 years and during each pregnancy.
Herpes zoster	(Preferred) RZV 2 doses at ≥50 years
Pneumococcal conjugate (PCV20 or PCV 15 followed by PPSV23)	One dose at ≥65 years.
Pneumococcal polysaccharide (PPSV23)	One dose at ≥65 years.
Note: Adults may need to receive the MMR, hepatitis A and B, meningococcal vaccines, HPV (females through age 26 and males through age 21), and varicella vaccines if they did not receive or complete the recommended vaccinations as children. Those traveling outside of the United States may require additional vaccines 6 weeks before travel, depending on the destination.	

Personalized Medicine

Key Pharmacokinetic Parameters

CL	Volume of blood/plasma cleared of a drug in a specified period of time. CL_{int} = intrinsic clearance.
C	Concentration
A	Amount of drug in the body
F (%)	Bioavailability of a drug. F_{po} – oral bioavailability
V_d	Volume of distribution or the amount of a drug in the body and its concentration in the blood or plasma. V_p = plasma volume, V_b = blood volume. V_c = volume or volume/amount.
$T_{1/2}$	Half life
f_u	Protein binding, f_{up} = fraction unbound in plasma, f_{ut} = fraction unbound in tissue.
Q	Organ blood flow, Q_H = hepatic blood flow
M	Metabolism
E	Excretion rate
BE	Bioequivalence
Ka	Absorption rate constant.

Therapeutic Index

The therapeutic index (T_i) indicates the degree of a drug's safety based on animal studies. The T_i is defined as the ratio of a drug's LD_{50} to its ED_{50}, where LD_{50} is the dose that is lethal to 50% of recipients and ED_{50} is the dose required to attain the desired (therapeutic) response in 50% of recipients.

$$T_i = LD_{50}/ED_{50}$$

A **high therapeutic index** indicates that the drug is relatively safe and a **low therapeutic index** indicates it is relatively unsafe. The relationship between the LD_{50} and the ED_{50} is important. For example, if the average therapeutic dose (ED_{50}) is much lower than the average lethal dose (LD_{50}), then the drug is likely relatively safe. Drugs with a low therapeutic index include anticholinergics because of a small difference in dose between LD_{50} and ED_{50}. Other drugs with a low therapeutic index include digoxin, lithium, aminoglycosides, cyclosporine, warfarin, carbamazepine, phenytoin, phenobarbital, theophylline, digitalis glycosides, flecainide, and rifampin.

Role of Pharmacogenomics in Producing Individualized Drug Therapy

Pharmacogenomics utilizes the information from molecular genetic tests to aid in diagnosis and treatment of disease with precision medicine that is individualized to meet the patient's distinct needs. Pharmacogenomics is the study of the way in which genes affect an individual's response to drug treatment. This information can help to produce drugs that cause fewer adverse effects and to predict the drugs that will be most effective. Genome-side association studies have helped to identify genetic abnormalities associated with different diseases. About 1800 genes have been identified with different diseases and only a small percentage have FDA-approved drugs for treatment. Over 1200 FDA-approved drugs target proteins associated with genes. As more and more genetic markers are identified, the research into development of precision medicine becomes more important because even the same disease in different individuals may be expressed differently. This may explain why current medications work well for some individuals but not others.

Loading Dose, Maintenance Dose, and Replacement Dose

Loading dose is an initial dose that is given to a patient to reach therapeutic levels of the drug rapidly, before the dose is tapered off to normal levels. Depends on the particular drug. A loading dose is common for anti-seizure medications, anticoagulants and some antibiotics. **Maintenance dose** is the minimum dose of a drug that is needed after initial loading dose to maintain an effective therapeutic level in the blood stream. **Replacement dose** is the dose administered as replacement of a missed dose of a drug. A replacement dose depends on a particular drug and may or may not be necessary.

Evidence-Based Practice

Evidence Based Medicine

Evidence based medicine has become a staple of modern healthcare. For this reason, primary literature is a valuable asset in the hospital setting. A pharmacist has the important role of keeping physicians informed of new medical findings and techniques that can be used to treat a particular patient. This use of evidence-based medicine is simultaneously a blessing and a bane of healthcare. It can keep the healthcare team on top of the newest trends in healthcare and can give ideas of reasonably safe approaches to treating the patients. Unfortunately, evidence-based medicine can also lead to stagnation. If a physician and a healthcare team rely solely on evidence-based medicine, this leaves little room for creativity and adaptation, which are often necessary when dealing with any particular patient. Like any research or therapy, medicine should be based both on previous used techniques and creative therapy (within reason).

Internet Sources of Evidence Based Medicine

The internet has provided an incredible means of achieving articles and data to support both research and evidence based medicine, linking to both primary and secondary scientific literature for both basic science and clinical studies.

- The Food and Drug Administration: fda.gov
- The Cochrane database, healthcare research review: cochrane.org
- PubMeb, huge repository of biomedical literature: pubmed.ncbi.nlm.nih.gov
- NatMed, natural medicines database: naturalmedicines.therapeuticresearch.com

Classes of Medical Literature

There are **three classes of medical literature**: primary, secondary and tertiary.

- **Primary literature** consists of original peer-reviewed scientific and medical articles, case reports and clinical trials that are published in reputable scientific journals.
- **Secondary literature** consists of abstracts, quick summaries and guides to primary literature. Secondary literature is often connected to primary literature and is often part of scientific journals, used to get an idea of what a paper is about before spending time actually reading it. Secondary literature is often an indicator of yet to be published data as well.
- **Tertiary literature** consists of review articles and textbooks. These literature types are summaries of primary literature and can be read to get an overall feel for a specific topic without usually going through all the data that was published on the topic. Additionally, tertiary literature often consists of common accepted knowledge in the medical or scientific field and does not necessarily need to be peer-reviewed.

Reliability and Validity in Evaluating Drug Research

In **drug research**, both reliability and validity of research findings must be assessed:

- **Reliability** refers to how consistently the measurement technique is able to measure the concept of interest. For example, if a measurement is taken at different times and the results are similar, this helps establish reliability. Reliability testing may be carried out to determine the degree of random error that can occur and how stable the results are over time. Equivalence compares two different measurements to determine if the findings are similar. A measure may be assessed globally or by unit of information.
- **Validity** refers to whether a measurement technique actually measures that which is intended and has accuracy (measures objectives precisely), utility (provides formative and summative results), and relevance (provides meaningful results). Content-validity determines whether all appropriate elements are measured, especially important in the development of drugs as overlooked parameters may have serious implications.

Criteria Needed for Medicare to Cover Clinical Trials

For **Medicare to cover clinical trials** including costs of conventional (normal) care and other drugs, certain characteristics must be met:

1. Patients must be 65 years or older.
2. Clinical trials cannot be for cosmetic purposes.
3. The clinical trial must have a specific therapeutic intent such as research for a specific treatment of a disease.
4. The patient must have distinct measurable symptoms for the disease in which the clinical trial is attempting to study and treat.

Stages of Clinical Trials

Described below are the three stages of clinical trials necessary for the FDA to approve a drug for human use as well as phase IV trials:

- **Phase I trials**: First human studies performed after successful preclinical animal studies of a given compound has shown some benefit. Phase I trials involve a small group of healthy volunteers to determine the toxicity and metabolism of the drug.

- **Phase II trials**: Provided to a larger population, the therapeutic efficacy and the required therapeutic dose of the drug are assessed. Safety assessment studies are continued during this time as well.
- **Phase III trials**: Performed to assess the effectiveness of the newly developed drug, in an unbiased controlled environment. Drug is tested in double blind study, in which test subjects are given either a placebo (a fake drug) or the drug being tested. The exact nature of the drug given to patients during the trial is hidden from both patient and physician. This is done to remove any possible bias during the experiments. If approved by the FDA, the drug can be put on the market.
- **Phase IV trials**: Post market safety surveillance. Companies that developed the new drug must monitor the drug's safety and efficacy in the larger population of patients and assess any possible long-term toxicity that the drug might possess.

NCE and NME

An **NCE (new chemical entity)** and **NME (new molecular entity)** are compounds, which have been developed and show therapeutic potential against a particular disease state or target in preclinical trials, but have not yet been studied in humans. As defined by the Food and Drug Administration, and NCE and NME, is a compound by which the region of the molecule responsible for the physiological changes or effects has not been approved by the FDA. Development of an NCE or NME is one of the first steps in drug development. Once preclinical trials are completed, the next step in drug development would be to begin studying the effects of the compounds on humans in phase I, phase II, and phase III clinical trials. If all goes well, following FDA approval, the compound can go to market.

Placebo Response

The placebo response is a phenomenon of clinical trials, in which pharmacologically inert sugar pills or other compounds that are used as controls, shows apparent beneficial biological effects. It is thought that the placebo drugs have this apparent beneficial response for numerous reasons, such as doctors, who do want their patients to feel better, inadvertently and subconsciously skew the data. Additionally, patients who feel that they might be receiving the experimental drug rather than an inert compound may feel they are feeling better due to a rather strong power of suggestion. The exact reason for a placebo response, however, is not entirely understood.

Nocebo Response

The nocebo response is the counterpart to the placebo response. It is not a term that is used as frequently as the placebo response. Nocebo is a pharmacologically inert compound that leads to apparent unwanted side effects. Some causes of the nocebo effect can be possible allergies to the fillers used in making the nocebo compound. It is thought that the nocebo response may have a more psychological basis, in that the patients could be using the power of suggestion (worrying too much) to make themselves sicker. The exact reason for a nocebo response, however, is not entirely understood.

FPGEE Practice Test

1. What are the primary functions that serotonin regulates? (Select ALL that apply).

A. Intestinal movements.
B. Mood and appetite.
C. Vasoconstriction and memory formation.
D. Sleep regulation.

2. What is the mechanism of action for acyclovir?

A. Interference with the function of viral M2 protein
B. Inhibition of pyrophosphate binding on virus-specific deoxyribonucleic acid (DNA) polymerases
C. Inhibition of DNA polymerase and incorporation into and termination of viral DNA
D. Reduction of viral replication and activity by inhibition of fusion between the plasma membrane and viral envelope

3. What is the volume of distribution (Vd) for aminoglycosides in a healthy adult?

A. 0.1–0.2 L/kg
B. 0.2–0.3 L/kg
C. 0.3–0.4 L/kg
D. 8 L

4. What is the infusion rate for dopamine at a concentration of 1.6 mg/mL being administered at 15 mcg/kg/min to a premature neonate weighing 1767 grams? (Constructed Response: Answer must be numeric; round the final answer to the nearest <u>WHOLE</u> number.)

5. Which of the following is an important counseling point for a patient taking rifampin?

A. Take rifampin with food
B. Do not take rifampin at the same time as antacids or milk
C. Rifampin may discolor urine, feces, tears, sweat, saliva, and soft contact lenses
D. Rifampin may cause dizziness

6. Which of the following chemotherapeutic agents acts by inhibiting dihydrofolate reductase and interfering with DNA synthesis, repair, and cellular reproduction?

A. Methotrexate
B. Cyclophosphamide
C. Mitoxantrone
D. Bleomycin

7. What is the meaning of the term "pharmacodynamics"?

A. The study of the effects of the body on medications (absorption, distribution, metabolism, and elimination)
B. The study of the influence of genetic variation on drug response
C. The study of the effects of drugs in large groups of people
D. The study of the effects of medications on the body (mechanisms of action)

8. A tobramycin blood level of 30.2 mcg/mL is drawn at 2:14 pm. A second level, drawn at 9:58 pm, is 2 mcg/mL. Approximately what is the half-life of the tobramycin? (Constructed Response: Answer must be numeric; round the final answer to the nearest WHOLE number.)

9. The type of insulin that forms a precipitate when injected into subcutaneous fat due to its acidic pH is which of the following?

A. Insulin glargine
B. Insulin lispro
C. Insulin aspart
D. Insulin detemir

10. Which of the following is a common viral capsid arrangement? (Select ALL that apply.)

A. Polyhedral
B. Helical
C. Binal
D. Spiral

11. Several injectable medications are available in preservative-free "pediatric formulations" that do not contain benzyl alcohol. Benzyl alcohol is omitted from these formulations because it causes which of the following conditions?

A. Fanconi syndrome
B. Agranulocytosis
C. Gasping syndrome
D. Congenital central hypoventilation syndrome (CCHS)

12. Which of the following are stated by pharmacists as a barrier for patient counseling? (Select ALL that apply.)

A. Poor response from patients
B. No ability to charge professional fee
C. Inadequate knowledge
D. Reduced patient compliance

13. Which of the following groups is most likely to use complementary/alternative medication therapies?

A. Asians
B. African Americans
C. Native Americans
D. Latinos

14. Which of the following is a common resistance mechanism for tetracyclines?

A. Ribosomal protection
B. Beta-lactamases
C. Target-site modifications
D. Enzyme target changes

15. The isoxazolyl group on the side chain of the penicillin nucleus of dicloxacillin (shown below) provides which of the following?

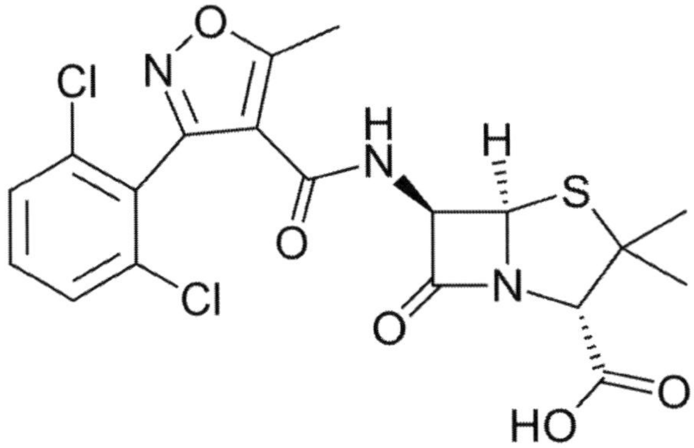

A. Activity against *Pseudomonas aeruginosa*
B. Resistance to beta-lactamases
C. Reduced incidence of diarrhea
D. Inability to bind to penicillin-binding proteins

16. Which of the following terms refers to an injection directly into the brain?

A. Intrathecal
B. Intraventricular
C. Intraosseous
D. Intraparenteral

17. Which component of a prescription contains instructions to the pharmacist regarding how to prepare a medication or the form of the medication?

A. Superscription
B. Inscription
C. Subscription
D. Sig

18. Which of the following muscles is commonly used for intramuscular injection? (Select ALL that apply.)

A. Gastrocnemius
B. Gluteus medius
C. Vastus lateralis
D. Deltoid

19. Which of the following is a symptom of aminoglycoside toxicity?

A. Gait instability
B. Increased liver function tests (LFTs)
C. Bradycardia
D. Ecchymosis

20. Which of the following is the most common reason that a patient stops patronizing a particular pharmacy?

A. Lower prices elsewhere
B. Relocation (the patient moves away)
C. Perceived employee indifference
D. Patient death

21. Which of the following herbal supplements taken concomitantly with warfarin may result in decreased warfarin plasma concentrations?

A. Echinacea
B. *Plantago*
C. Valerian root
D. St. John's wort

22. The atomic weights of magnesium, sulfur, and oxygen are 24, 32, and 16, respectively. A solution contains 3 g of MgSO4. How many milliequivalents (mEq) of MgSO4 are present in the solution? (Constructed Response: Answer must be numeric; round the final answer to the nearest <u>WHOLE</u> number.)

23. Which of the following is an essential amino acid?

A. Tyrosine
B. Asparagine
C. Phenylalanine
D. Cysteine

24. Excess buildup of iron due to blood transfusions can be treated parenterally with which of the following medications?

A. Deferasirox
B. Deferiprone
C. Defibrotide
D. Deferoxamine

25. Which of the following medications exhibits a "first-dose effect"?

A. Verapamil
B. Enalapril
C. Terazosin
D. Atenolol

26. Why is epinephrine added to some formulations of lidocaine (e.g., Xylocaine with epinephrine)?

A. To prolong the effect of the lidocaine
B. To shorten the effect of the lidocaine
C. To minimize the side effects of the lidocaine
D. To prevent an allergic reaction to the lidocaine

27. Peak plasma levels of which of the following hormones will be reached during ovulation?

A. Estrogen and progesterone
B. Follicle-stimulating hormone (FSH) and luteinizing hormone (LH)
C. Progesterone and LH
D. Estrogen and FSH

28. A total parenteral nutrition (TPN) bag with a volume of 1440 mL has a final concentration of potassium acetate of 55 mEq/L. How many 20-mL vials of 2 mEq/mL potassium acetate must be used to compound the TPN? (Constructed Response: Answer must be numeric; round the final answer to the nearest WHOLE number.)

29. What does it mean when a patient is instructed to be NPO?

A. Nothing by mouth
B. No rectal products
C. No parenteral injections
D. No topical applications

30. What is the bioavailability of a medication that is administered intravenously?

A. 12.5%
B. 25%
C. 50%
D. 100%

31. Which of the following is a requirement for medications to be considered therapeutically equivalent by the Food and Drug Administration (FDA)? (Select ALL that apply.)

A. Same dosage form
B. Same active ingredient
C. Same excipients
D. Same route of administration

32. Which of the following medications should be administered at least one hour before or four to six hours after other medications?

A. Amoxicillin
B. Famotidine
C. Cholestyramine
D. Levothyroxine

33. Which of the following is a B vitamin? (Select ALL that apply.)

A. Leucine
B. Thiamine
C. Folic acid
D. Pyridoxine

34. Which of the following salts is an injectable form of erythromycin?

A. Erythromycin stearate
B. Erythromycin ethylsuccinate
C. Erythromycin lactobionate
D. Erythromycin estolate

35. How does pantoprazole (Protonix) reduce gastric-acid secretion?

A. Histamine blockade
B. Proton-pump inhibition
C. Acetylcholine blockade
D. Buffering

36. Which of the following anti-infective agents is LEAST likely to cause *Clostridioides difficile* colitis?

A. Erythromycin
B. Clindamycin
C. Tetracycline
D. Metronidazole

37. Which of the following strategies enhances calcium and phosphate solubility in total parenteral nutrition (TPN) formulations?

A. Raising the pH
B. Increasing the temperature
C. Adding L-cysteine
D. Decreasing the amino-acid concentration

38. Rizatriptan (Maxalt) is used in the treatment of which of the following conditions?

A. Migraine headaches
B. Depression
C. Hypertension
D. Arrhythmia

39. Which of the following agents is most similar to chlorthalidone?

A. Furosemide
B. Metolazone
C. Hydrochlorothiazide
D. Ethacrynic acid

40. A physician describes a patient as being thrombocytopenic. What does this term mean?

A. Decreased number of platelets in the blood
B. Increased number of platelets in the blood
C. Decreased number of white blood cells (WBCs) in the blood
D. Increased number of WBCs in the blood

41. A patient reports taking the following medications: pancrelipase (Creon), dornase alfa (Pulmozyme), salmeterol/fluticasone (Advair Diskus), inhaled tobramycin (Tobi), vitamins A, D, E, K (ADEKs), and lansoprazole (Prevacid). What medical condition does this patient have?

A. Sickle-cell disease
B. Cystic fibrosis
C. Muscular dystrophy
D. Cerebral palsy

42. Which of the following medications is highly protein bound? (Select ALL that apply.)

A. Warfarin
B. Phenytoin
C. Valproic acid
D. Ketamine

43. A patient complains of dry mouth (xerostomia). Which of the following medications is most likely to cause this side effect?

A. Doxepin
B. Famotidine
C. Dabigatran
D. Enalapril

44. Which of the following medications should be taken with food?

A. Indomethacin
B. Levofloxacin
C. Enalapril
D. Tamsulosin

45. Which of the following antibiotics uses concentration-dependent killing?

A. Meropenem
B. Cephalexin
C. Ciprofloxacin
D. Clindamycin

46. Which of the following medications should be avoided in a patient with a sulfa allergy?

A. Anastrozole
B. Dapsone
C. Finasteride
D. Amoxicillin

47. Which of the following antiemetics carries a black box warning regarding the risks of severe tissue injury, including gangrene, associated with its administration?

A. Ondansetron (Zofran)
B. Droperidol (Inapsine)
C. Lorazepam (Ativan)
D. Promethazine (Phenergan)

48. Which of the following chemotherapeutic agents is an alkylator?

A. Docetaxel
B. Cisplatin
C. Vinorelbine
D. Idarubicin

49. A pharmacist receives a prescription with the sig, "3 gtt au qid." By what route will this medication be given?

A. Left ear
B. Left eye
C. Both eyes
D. Both ears

50. Once a drug is at steady state, when should a serum trough level of a medication be drawn?

A. Anytime during the dosing interval
B. Immediately after the dose has been administered
C. In the middle of the dosing interval
D. Immediately prior to dose administration

Answer Key and Explanations

1. A, B, and D: Mood, appetite, intestinal movements, and sleep are the primary functions that serotonin regulates. Certain antidepressants [e.g., selective serotonin reuptake inhibitors (SSRIs)], antimigraine agents (e.g., triptans), and antiemetics (e.g., 5-HT_3-receptor antagonists) are examples of drugs that target the serotonin system.

2. C: Acyclovir's mechanism of action is competitive inhibition of DNA polymerase and incorporation into and termination of viral DNA. Viral and cellular enzymes convert acyclovir to a triphosphate analog, which is incorporated into viral DNA and irreversibly bound, thereby terminating growing viral DNA chains.

3. B: The volume of distribution (Vd) in healthy adults is about 0.25 L/kg. The Vd is increased in patients with increased extracellular fluid (higher total body water content) such as pediatric patients, cystic fibrosis patients, or patients with ascites. The Vd is decreased in patients with decreased extracellular fluid (lower total body water content), such as in patients with dehydration.

4. $\frac{15 \text{ mcg}}{\text{kg} \times \text{min}} \times 1767 \text{ g} \times \frac{\text{kg}}{1000 \text{ g}} \times \frac{60 \text{ min}}{\text{hr}} \times \frac{\text{mL}}{1.6 \text{ mg}} \times \frac{\text{mg}}{1000 \text{ mcg}} = \mathbf{1\ mL/hr}$

5. C: Rifampin has an intense red color and may discolor urine, feces, tears, sweat, saliva, and soft contact lenses. Patients may mistake the red color as blood, so they should be counseled about the possible discoloration of bodily fluids. Food decreases the absorption of rifampin, so the drug should be taken on an empty stomach; antacids do not affect absorption.

6. A: Methotrexate acts by inhibiting dihydrofolate reductase and interfering with DNA synthesis, repair, and cellular reproduction. Dihydrofolate reductase converts dihydrofolate to tetrahydrofolate, which is necessary for purine synthesis in healthy cells as well as cancerous cells. Therefore, methotrexate can cause profound neutropenia unless leucovorin (folinic acid) rescue is administered concomitantly.

7. D: Pharmacodynamics is the study of the effects of medications on the body (mechanisms of action). The study of the effects of the body on medications (absorption, distribution, metabolism, elimination) is called pharmacokinetics. Pharmacogenomics is the study of the influence of genetic variations on drug response, and the study of the effects of drugs in large groups of people is called pharmacoepidemiology.

8. $\frac{30.2 \text{ mcg/mL}}{2} = 15.1 \text{ mcg/mL}$ $\frac{15.1 \text{ mcg/mL}}{2} = 7.55 \text{ mcg/mL}$ $\frac{7.55 \text{ mcg/mL}}{2} = 3.755 \text{ mcg/mL}$
$\frac{3.755 \text{ mcg/mL}}{2} = 1.8875 \text{ mcg/mL}$

- 30. 2 mcg/mL is reduced to 2 mcg/mL in approximately four half-lives.
- 9:58 pm is approximately eight hours after 2:14 pm.
- $\frac{8 \text{ hours}}{4 \text{ half lives}}$ = **Two hours per half-life.**

9. A: Insulin glargine precipitates when injected into subcutaneous fat due to its acidic pH, thereby forming a depot, which is responsible for its prolonged absorption and constant concentration/time profile.

10. A, B, and C: Viruses consist of nucleic acid surrounded by protein. Repeating protein subunits form the outer protein, or capsid. The arrangement of the capsid is polyhedral, helical, or binal, and this determines the form of the virus.

11. C: Gasping syndrome in a neonate is caused by the newborn's inability to metabolize benzyl alcohol, and it is characterized by metabolic acidosis, seizures, neurologic deterioration, gasping respirations, bradycardia, hypotension, and death.

12. A, B, and C: Reduced patient compliance is not stated by pharmacists to be a reason for patient counseling; *improved* patient compliance is stated by pharmacists to be a reason **for** providing patient counseling. Poor response from patients, no ability to charge a professional fee, and inadequate knowledge are all stated by pharmacists as barriers for patient counseling.

13. C: Native Americans are most likely to use complementary/alternative medication therapies of the groups listed. Examples of complementary and alternative medications (CAMs) include acupuncture, biofeedback, hypnosis, meditation, massage, and herbal medications. Back pain is the most common condition for which CAMs are used in adult populations.

14. A: Tetracycline efflux, ribosomal protection, and tetracycline modification are the three mechanisms of tetracycline resistance. Beta-lactamases target beta-lactam antibiotics; target-site modifications are seen in beta-lactams, vancomycin, and quinolones; and enzyme target change resistance is seen in quinolones and sulfonamides.

15. B: The isoxazolyl group prevents hydrolysis of the beta-lactam ring by penicillinase, thereby producing resistance to the beta-lactamase. Other examples of beta-lactamase-resistant penicillins are cloxacillin, methicillin, nafcillin, and oxacillin.

16. B: The ventricular system in the brain consists of the left and right lateral ventricles and the third and fourth ventricles. The ventricles contain cerebrospinal fluid (CSF), which acts as a cushion and provides buoyancy for the brain. Antiepileptics, chemotherapy, and pain medication are examples of drugs that can be advantageously injected intraventricularly by providing a greater concentration of the medication at the desired site of action.

17. C: A prescription is comprised of seven parts (in Latin): *inscriptio, praepositio, prescriptio, subscriptio, singatura, nomen medici,* and *nomen aegroti*. The *subscriptio* (subscription) contains instructions to the pharmacist regarding how to prepare the medication or the amount of the medication to dispense (e.g., "#10 capsules").

18. B, C, and D: The gastrocnemius muscle is one of the calf muscles and is not commonly used for intramuscular injection. Intramuscular injections are generally given in the upper arm (the deltoid), one of the hip muscles (gluteus maximus, gluteus medius, or gluteus minimus), or the outside of the upper leg (the vastus lateralis).

19. A: Ototoxicity and nephrotoxicity are the most serious side effects of aminoglycosides because they can be permanent. Auditory and vestibular functions of the ear can be affected; thus, gait instability can be an indication of toxicity. Ototoxicity is caused by the accumulation of the drug in the perilymph and endolymph of the inner ear; half-lives of aminoglycosides in the ear are five to six times those of plasma.

20. C: The most common reason that a patient stops patronizing a particular pharmacy is due to perceived employee indifference. Patient counseling has been suggested to be a strategy for improving customer loyalty. In addition to preventing prescription errors, patient counseling can enhance the relationship between the patient and the pharmacist and improve patient compliance.

21. D: St. John's wort, marketed as an antidepressant, is a popular herbal medication that induces the cytochrome P450 isoenzymes CYP2C9 and CYP3A4; these isoenzymes are involved in the metabolism of warfarin. St. John's wort enhances the metabolism of warfarin, decreasing plasma concentrations and reducing the anticoagulant effect of warfarin.

22. Calculate the molecular weight (MW) of $MgSO_4$:

1. 24 g + 32 g + 4(16 g) = 120 g.
2. Calculate the equivalent weight (Eq):

   Eq = MW / valence* = 120 g/2 = 60 g (1 Eq of MgSO4 weighs 60 g).

1. *The valence of an element is equal to the number of electrons in its outer shell; a magnesium ion has a charge of +2, and a sulfate ion has a charge of −2, so the valence of $MgSO_4$ is 2.
2. Solve for the number of milliequivalents (mEq):

$$3\text{ g} \times \frac{1\text{ Eq}}{60\text{ g}} \times \frac{1000\text{ mEq}}{\text{Eq}} = \mathbf{50\ mEq}$$

23. C: An essential amino acid is one that cannot be synthesized by the body, so it must come from the diet. Phenylalanine is used in the synthesis of catecholamines. Patients with phenylketonuria (PKU) are unable to break down phenylalanine; this disorder can be treated by following a low-phenylalanine diet. Testing for this disorder is included in state screens, which are administered to newborns in all 50 states.

24. D: Deferoxamine mesylate is a chelator, which is used to treat iron overload. It binds to iron, which is then eliminated in the feces and urine. It is administered intravenously, subcutaneously, or intramuscularly. Deferasirox and deferiprone are chelators that are administered orally.

25. C: Terazosin and other alpha-adrenergic blockers can exhibit a first-dose effect, in which a patient experiences a sudden drop in blood pressure after taking the first dose; syncope can result when the patient rises from a lying or sitting position. Patients should be counseled about this phenomenon.

26. A: Epinephrine is added to lidocaine and other local anesthetics to prolong their effects. The half-life of lidocaine is very short; the epinephrine causes local vasoconstriction and reduces the rate of lidocaine removal to the area where it was injected.

27. B: At the time of ovulation, the concentrations of follicle-stimulating hormone (FSH) and luteinizing hormone (LH) reach their peaks. This corresponds with the release of the ovum and the thickening of the endometrial wall in preparation for implantation of the embryo.

28. $\frac{55\text{ mEq}}{\text{L}} \times \frac{1400\text{ mL}}{\text{bag}} \times \frac{1\text{ L}}{1000\text{ mL}} \times \frac{\text{mL}}{2\text{ mEq}} \times \frac{\text{vial}}{20\text{ mL}} = \frac{1.925\text{ vials}}{\text{bag}} = \mathbf{2\ vials\ to\ make\ 1\ bag}$

29. A: NPO is an abbreviation for the Latin term "*nil per os*." Translated, this means "nothing by mouth"; a patient should refrain from eating or drinking for the period of time specified by the prescriber. Patients are often instructed to remain NPO prior to undergoing certain medical tests or prior to surgery.

30. D: Bioavailability measures the amount of unchanged drug that reaches the systemic circulation. The bioavailability of a medication that is administered intravenously is 100% because it is being directly injected into the systemic circulation. Bioavailability is affected by absorption and the first-pass effect.

31. A, B, and D: For medications to be considered therapeutically equivalent by the Food and Drug Administration (FDA), they must share the same dosage form (e.g., capsule), the same active ingredient (e.g., hydrochlorothiazide), and the same route of administration (e.g., oral). However, they can have different excipients (fillers).

32. C: Cholestyramine is a bile acid sequestrant used to lower cholesterol by binding bile in the gastrointestinal tract and preventing its reabsorption. Cholestyramine can bind other medications before they are fully absorbed, so it is recommended to administer other medications one hour prior to or at least four hours after cholestyramine administration.

33. B, C, and D: Leucine is an amino acid. Thiamine (B_1), riboflavin (B_2), niacin (B_3), pantothenic acid (B_5), pyridoxine (B_6), biotin (B_7), folic acid (B_9), and cyanocobalamin (B_{12}) are the B vitamins. The B vitamins are water-soluble and are used for various functions by the body, including energy generation.

34. C: Erythromycin lactobionate is the injectable form of erythromycin; it is soluble in water. The stearate, ethylsuccinate, and estolate salts of erythromycin are poorly soluble in water, which make them unsuitable for intravenous administration.

35. B: Pantoprazole and other proton-pump inhibitors block gastric acid secretion of gastric parietal cells by inhibiting the H^+, K^+, ATPase pump. This system exchanges a hydrogen ion (H^+) from the cytoplasm of the parietal cell with one potassium ion (K^+) from the gastric lumen.

36. D: Pseudomembranous colitis occurs when other bacteria in the gut have been affected by antibiotics and an overgrowth of gram-positive Clostridioides difficile (commonly called C. diff) results. *C. diff* releases a toxin that inflames the lining of the colon and can cause abdominal cramping, bloody stools, and severe diarrhea; it can also lead to toxic megacolon. It is treated with oral vancomycin or intravenous or oral metronidazole. Fluoroquinolones, clindamycin, penicillins, and cephalosporins are frequently associated with the development of *C. diff.*

37. C: Inclusion of calcium and phosphate in TPN formulations is limited because of precipitation. Several factors influence the solubility of calcium and phosphate, including temperature, pH, amino-acid concentration, and inclusion of L-cysteine. Solubility of these components is increased at lower temperatures and a lower pH. Adding L-cysteine lowers the pH, thereby improving calcium–phosphate solubility.

38. A: Rizatriptan and other $5\text{-HT}_{1B/1D}$-receptor agonists are used in the treatment of migraine headaches. They have multiple mechanisms of action associated with activity at these receptors, including vasoconstriction of cerebral blood vessels, inhibition of the release of vasoactive neuropeptides by trigeminal nerves, and inhibition of nociceptive neurotransmission.

39. C: Hydrochlorothiazide is a thiazide diuretic. Chlorthalidone is similar in its mechanism of action, although it is slightly different structurally. Both act in the distal convoluted tubule to reduce sodium reabsorption, resulting in decreased exocellular fluid and plasma volume, thereby reducing blood pressure.

40. A: Thrombocytes are platelets, and the suffix *-penia* is Greek for "deficiency"; therefore, a lower than normal number of platelets in the blood is referred to as thrombocytopenia. The normal range for platelets is 150–450 x $10^3/\mu L$, so if a patient has platelets measuring less than $150{,}000/\mu L$, he or she is thrombocytopenic.

41. B: Cystic fibrosis (CF) is caused by a defect in the cystic fibrosis transmembrane conductance regulator (CFTR) gene, which controls the flow of water and salt into and out of cells. The result is thick, sticky mucus throughout the body, which can result in blockage. CF patients experience symptoms such as recurrent lung infections, clogged pancreatic ducts, malabsorption, nasal polyps, and sinus infections. Common medications taken by CF patients include pancreatic enzymes, proton-pump inhibitors (to aid in absorption of the enzymes), supplemental fat-soluble vitamins, bronchodilators, dornase alfa (Pulmozyme) (to cleave the DNA present in the mucus), and antibiotics that treat *Pseudomonas aeruginosa*.

42. A, B, and C: Some drugs bind to plasma proteins, which reduces the amount of drug available for interacting with receptors and producing pharmacological effects. The fraction of drug that is not bound to protein is what is being measured when sampling serum drug concentrations. Warfarin, phenytoin, and valproic acid are all highly protein bound.

43. A: Doxepin is a tricyclic antidepressant (TCA) that exhibits strong anticholinergic effects, including drowsiness, dry mouth (xerostomia), pupil dilation (mydriasis), urinary retention, and constipation. Desipramine (Norpramin) exhibits the fewest anticholinergic side effects of any of the TCAs.

44. A: Indomethacin is a nonsteroidal anti-inflammatory drug (NSAID). All NSAIDs can cause severe gastrointestinal (GI) effects, including bleeding, ulceration, and perforation of the stomach or intestines, but indomethacin is especially hard on the GI system. H_2-blockers or proton-pump inhibitors are often prescribed concomitantly with indomethacin for stomach protection.

45. C: The pharmacodynamic properties of fluoroquinolones (FQs) such as ciprofloxacin are such that maximizing concentration results in more extensive and faster killing of infectious organisms. This is commonly referred to as "concentration-dependent killing." Ketolides (e.g., telithromycin), aminoglycosides, and daptomycin also exhibit concentration-dependent killing.

46. B: Patients with allergies to sulfonamides have been shown to have cross-reactivity to dapsone. Though they are structurally different from dapsone, the sulfonamides and dapsone share a mechanism of action (inhibition of bacterial dihydrofolic acid synthesis). Dapsone is commonly used for skin conditions, leprosy, and *Pneumocystis jiroveci* pneumonia prophylaxis.

47. D: The black box warning for promethazine states that "Irritation and damage can result from perivascular extravasation, unintentional intra-arterial injection, and intraneuronal or perineuronal infiltration. Adverse reactions include burning, pain, thrombophlebitis, tissue necrosis, and gangrene. In some cases, surgical intervention (including fasciotomy, skin graft, and/or amputation) has been required." The FDA recommends deep intramuscular injection as the preferred route for this medication.

48. B: Alkylating agents add an alkyl group to deoxyribonucleic acid (DNA) strands of cancer cells, preventing the proteins encoded by the DNA to link properly, thereby causing breaks in the DNA strands and cell death. Alkylating agents are cell-cycle nonspecific, meaning that they have activity during all phases of the cell cycle (G_0, G_1, S, G_2, and M). Cisplatin is an example of an alkylating agent.

49. D: AU stands for the Latin *auris uterque*, meaning both ears. "Left ear" is abbreviated as AS (*auris sinistra*); "right ear" is abbreviated as AD (*auris dextra*). "Left eye" is abbreviated as OS (*oculus sinister*); "right eye" is abbreviated as OD (*oculus dexter*). The term "both eyes" is abbreviated as OU (*oculus uterque* or *oculi uterque*).

50. D: The "trough" is intended to represent the point at which the least amount of medication is present in the systemic circulation; therefore, the most appropriate sampling time for a trough level is just before the dose is due.

How to Overcome Test Anxiety

Just the thought of taking a test is enough to make most people a little nervous. A test is an important event that can have a long-term impact on your future, so it's important to take it seriously and it's natural to feel anxious about performing well. But just because anxiety is normal, that doesn't mean that it's helpful in test taking, or that you should simply accept it as part of your life. Anxiety can have a variety of effects. These effects can be mild, like making you feel slightly nervous, or severe, like blocking your ability to focus or remember even a simple detail.

If you experience test anxiety—whether severe or mild—it's important to know how to beat it. To discover this, first you need to understand what causes test anxiety.

Causes of Test Anxiety

While we often think of anxiety as an uncontrollable emotional state, it can actually be caused by simple, practical things. One of the most common causes of test anxiety is that a person does not feel adequately prepared for their test. This feeling can be the result of many different issues such as poor study habits or lack of organization, but the most common culprit is time management. Starting to study too late, failing to organize your study time to cover all of the material, or being distracted while you study will mean that you're not well prepared for the test. This may lead to cramming the night before, which will cause you to be physically and mentally exhausted for the test. Poor time management also contributes to feelings of stress, fear, and hopelessness as you realize you are not well prepared but don't know what to do about it.

Other times, test anxiety is not related to your preparation for the test but comes from unresolved fear. This may be a past failure on a test, or poor performance on tests in general. It may come from comparing yourself to others who seem to be performing better or from the stress of living up to expectations. Anxiety may be driven by fears of the future—how failure on this test would affect your educational and career goals. These fears are often completely irrational, but they can still negatively impact your test performance.

Elements of Test Anxiety

As mentioned earlier, test anxiety is considered to be an emotional state, but it has physical and mental components as well. Sometimes you may not even realize that you are suffering from test anxiety until you notice the physical symptoms. These can include trembling hands, rapid heartbeat, sweating, nausea, and tense muscles. Extreme anxiety may lead to fainting or vomiting. Obviously, any of these symptoms can have a negative impact on testing. It is important to recognize them as soon as they begin to occur so that you can address the problem before it damages your performance.

The mental components of test anxiety include trouble focusing and inability to remember learned information. During a test, your mind is on high alert, which can help you recall information and stay focused for an extended period of time. However, anxiety interferes with your mind's natural processes, causing you to blank out, even on the questions you know well. The strain of testing during anxiety makes it difficult to stay focused, especially on a test that may take several hours. Extreme anxiety can take a huge mental toll, making it difficult not only to recall test information but even to understand the test questions or pull your thoughts together.

Effects of Test Anxiety

Test anxiety is like a disease—if left untreated, it will get progressively worse. Anxiety leads to poor performance, and this reinforces the feelings of fear and failure, which in turn lead to poor performances on subsequent tests. It can grow from a mild nervousness to a crippling condition. If allowed to progress, test anxiety can have a big impact on your schooling, and consequently on your future.

Test anxiety can spread to other parts of your life. Anxiety on tests can become anxiety in any stressful situation, and blanking on a test can turn into panicking in a job situation. But fortunately, you don't have to let anxiety rule your testing and determine your grades. There are a number of relatively simple steps you can take to move past anxiety and function normally on a test and in the rest of life.

Physical Steps for Beating Test Anxiety

While test anxiety is a serious problem, the good news is that it can be overcome. It doesn't have to control your ability to think and remember information. While it may take time, you can begin taking steps today to beat anxiety.

Just as your first hint that you may be struggling with anxiety comes from the physical symptoms, the first step to treating it is also physical. Rest is crucial for having a clear, strong mind. If you are tired, it is much easier to give in to anxiety. But if you establish good sleep habits, your body and mind will be ready to perform optimally, without the strain of exhaustion. Additionally, sleeping well helps you to retain information better, so you're more likely to recall the answers when you see the test questions.

Getting good sleep means more than going to bed on time. It's important to allow your brain time to relax. Take study breaks from time to time so it doesn't get overworked, and don't study right before bed. Take time to rest your mind before trying to rest your body, or you may find it difficult to fall asleep.

Along with sleep, other aspects of physical health are important in preparing for a test. Good nutrition is vital for good brain function. Sugary foods and drinks may give a burst of energy but this burst is followed by a crash, both physically and emotionally. Instead, fuel your body with protein and vitamin-rich foods.

Also, drink plenty of water. Dehydration can lead to headaches and exhaustion, especially if your brain is already under stress from the rigors of the test. Particularly if your test is a long one, drink water during the breaks. And if possible, take an energy-boosting snack to eat between sections.

Along with sleep and diet, a third important part of physical health is exercise. Maintaining a steady workout schedule is helpful, but even taking 5-minute study breaks to walk can help get your blood pumping faster and clear your head. Exercise also releases endorphins, which contribute to a positive feeling and can help combat test anxiety.

When you nurture your physical health, you are also contributing to your mental health. If your body is healthy, your mind is much more likely to be healthy as well. So take time to rest, nourish your body with healthy food and water, and get moving as much as possible. Taking these physical steps will make you stronger and more able to take the mental steps necessary to overcome test anxiety.

Mental Steps for Beating Test Anxiety

Working on the mental side of test anxiety can be more challenging, but as with the physical side, there are clear steps you can take to overcome it. As mentioned earlier, test anxiety often stems from lack of preparation, so the obvious solution is to prepare for the test. Effective studying may be the most important weapon you have for beating test anxiety, but you can and should employ several other mental tools to combat fear.

First, boost your confidence by reminding yourself of past success—tests or projects that you aced. If you're putting as much effort into preparing for this test as you did for those, there's no reason you should expect to fail here. Work hard to prepare; then trust your preparation.

Second, surround yourself with encouraging people. It can be helpful to find a study group, but be sure that the people you're around will encourage a positive attitude. If you spend time with others who are anxious or cynical, this will only contribute to your own anxiety. Look for others who are motivated to study hard from a desire to succeed, not from a fear of failure.

Third, reward yourself. A test is physically and mentally tiring, even without anxiety, and it can be helpful to have something to look forward to. Plan an activity following the test, regardless of the outcome, such as going to a movie or getting ice cream.

When you are taking the test, if you find yourself beginning to feel anxious, remind yourself that you know the material. Visualize successfully completing the test. Then take a few deep, relaxing breaths and return to it. Work through the questions carefully but with confidence, knowing that you are capable of succeeding.

Developing a healthy mental approach to test taking will also aid in other areas of life. Test anxiety affects more than just the actual test—it can be damaging to your mental health and even contribute to depression. It's important to beat test anxiety before it becomes a problem for more than testing.

Study Strategy

Being prepared for the test is necessary to combat anxiety, but what does being prepared look like? You may study for hours on end and still not feel prepared. What you need is a strategy for test prep. The next few pages outline our recommended steps to help you plan out and conquer the challenge of preparation.

Step 1: Scope Out the Test

Learn everything you can about the format (multiple choice, essay, etc.) and what will be on the test. Gather any study materials, course outlines, or sample exams that may be available. Not only will this help you to prepare, but knowing what to expect can help to alleviate test anxiety.

Step 2: Map Out the Material

Look through the textbook or study guide and make note of how many chapters or sections it has. Then divide these over the time you have. For example, if a book has 15 chapters and you have five days to study, you need to cover three chapters each day. Even better, if you have the time, leave an extra day at the end for overall review after you have gone through the material in depth.

If time is limited, you may need to prioritize the material. Look through it and make note of which sections you think you already have a good grasp on, and which need review. While you are studying, skim quickly through the familiar sections and take more time on the challenging parts.

Write out your plan so you don't get lost as you go. Having a written plan also helps you feel more in control of the study, so anxiety is less likely to arise from feeling overwhelmed at the amount to cover.

Step 3: Gather Your Tools

Decide what study method works best for you. Do you prefer to highlight in the book as you study and then go back over the highlighted portions? Or do you type out notes of the important information? Or is it helpful to make flashcards that you can carry with you? Assemble the pens, index cards, highlighters, post-it notes, and any other materials you may need so you won't be distracted by getting up to find things while you study.

If you're having a hard time retaining the information or organizing your notes, experiment with different methods. For example, try color-coding by subject with colored pens, highlighters, or post-it notes. If you learn better by hearing, try recording yourself reading your notes so you can listen while in the car, working out, or simply sitting at your desk. Ask a friend to quiz you from your flashcards, or try teaching someone the material to solidify it in your mind.

Step 4: Create Your Environment

It's important to avoid distractions while you study. This includes both the obvious distractions like visitors and the subtle distractions like an uncomfortable chair (or a too-comfortable couch that makes you want to fall asleep). Set up the best study environment possible: good lighting and a comfortable work area. If background music helps you focus, you may want to turn it on, but otherwise keep the room quiet. If you are using a computer to take notes, be sure you don't have any other windows open, especially applications like social media, games, or anything else that could distract you. Silence your phone and turn off notifications. Be sure to keep water close by so you stay hydrated while you study (but avoid unhealthy drinks and snacks).

Also, take into account the best time of day to study. Are you freshest first thing in the morning? Try to set aside some time then to work through the material. Is your mind clearer in the afternoon or evening? Schedule your study session then. Another method is to study at the same time of day that you will take the test, so that your brain gets used to working on the material at that time and will be ready to focus at test time.

Step 5: Study!

Once you have done all the study preparation, it's time to settle into the actual studying. Sit down, take a few moments to settle your mind so you can focus, and begin to follow your study plan. Don't give in to distractions or let yourself procrastinate. This is your time to prepare so you'll be ready to fearlessly approach the test. Make the most of the time and stay focused.

Of course, you don't want to burn out. If you study too long you may find that you're not retaining the information very well. Take regular study breaks. For example, taking five minutes out of every hour to walk briskly, breathing deeply and swinging your arms, can help your mind stay fresh.

As you get to the end of each chapter or section, it's a good idea to do a quick review. Remind yourself of what you learned and work on any difficult parts. When you feel that you've mastered the material, move on to the next part. At the end of your study session, briefly skim through your notes again.

But while review is helpful, cramming last minute is NOT. If at all possible, work ahead so that you won't need to fit all your study into the last day. Cramming overloads your brain with more information than it can process and retain, and your tired mind may struggle to recall even previously learned information when it is overwhelmed with last-minute study. Also, the urgent nature of cramming and the stress placed on your brain contribute to anxiety. You'll be more likely to go to the test feeling unprepared and having trouble thinking clearly.

So don't cram, and don't stay up late before the test, even just to review your notes at a leisurely pace. Your brain needs rest more than it needs to go over the information again. In fact, plan to finish your studies by noon or early afternoon the day before the test. Give your brain the rest of the day to relax or focus on other things, and get a good night's sleep. Then you will be fresh for the test and better able to recall what you've studied.

Step 6: Take a Practice Test

Many courses offer sample tests, either online or in the study materials. This is an excellent resource to check whether you have mastered the material, as well as to prepare for the test format and environment.

Check the test format ahead of time: the number of questions, the type (multiple choice, free response, etc.), and the time limit. Then create a plan for working through them. For example, if you have 30 minutes to take a 60-question test, your limit is 30 seconds per question. Spend less time on the questions you know well so that you can take more time on the difficult ones.

If you have time to take several practice tests, take the first one open book, with no time limit. Work through the questions at your own pace and make sure you fully understand them. Gradually work up to taking a test under test conditions: sit at a desk with all study materials put away and set a timer. Pace yourself to make sure you finish the test with time to spare and go back to check your answers if you have time.

After each test, check your answers. On the questions you missed, be sure you understand why you missed them. Did you misread the question (tests can use tricky wording)? Did you forget the information? Or was it something you hadn't learned? Go back and study any shaky areas that the practice tests reveal.

Taking these tests not only helps with your grade, but also aids in combating test anxiety. If you're already used to the test conditions, you're less likely to worry about it, and working through tests until you're scoring well gives you a confidence boost. Go through the practice tests until you feel comfortable, and then you can go into the test knowing that you're ready for it.

Test Tips

On test day, you should be confident, knowing that you've prepared well and are ready to answer the questions. But aside from preparation, there are several test day strategies you can employ to maximize your performance.

First, as stated before, get a good night's sleep the night before the test (and for several nights before that, if possible). Go into the test with a fresh, alert mind rather than staying up late to study.

Try not to change too much about your normal routine on the day of the test. It's important to eat a nutritious breakfast, but if you normally don't eat breakfast at all, consider eating just a protein bar. If you're a coffee drinker, go ahead and have your normal coffee. Just make sure you time it so that the caffeine doesn't wear off right in the middle of your test. Avoid sugary beverages, and drink enough water to stay hydrated but not so much that you need a restroom break 10 minutes into the test. If your test isn't first thing in the morning, consider going for a walk or doing a light workout before the test to get your blood flowing.

Allow yourself enough time to get ready, and leave for the test with plenty of time to spare so you won't have the anxiety of scrambling to arrive in time. Another reason to be early is to select a good seat. It's helpful to sit away from doors and windows, which can be distracting. Find a good seat, get out your supplies, and settle your mind before the test begins.

When the test begins, start by going over the instructions carefully, even if you already know what to expect. Make sure you avoid any careless mistakes by following the directions.

Then begin working through the questions, pacing yourself as you've practiced. If you're not sure on an answer, don't spend too much time on it, and don't let it shake your confidence. Either skip it and come back later, or eliminate as many wrong answers as possible and guess among the remaining ones. Don't dwell on these questions as you continue—put them out of your mind and focus on what lies ahead.

Be sure to read all of the answer choices, even if you're sure the first one is the right answer. Sometimes you'll find a better one if you keep reading. But don't second-guess yourself if you do immediately know the answer. Your gut instinct is usually right. Don't let test anxiety rob you of the information you know.

If you have time at the end of the test (and if the test format allows), go back and review your answers. Be cautious about changing any, since your first instinct tends to be correct, but make sure you didn't misread any of the questions or accidentally mark the wrong answer choice. Look over any you skipped and make an educated guess.

At the end, leave the test feeling confident. You've done your best, so don't waste time worrying about your performance or wishing you could change anything. Instead, celebrate the successful completion of this test. And finally, use this test to learn how to deal with anxiety even better next time.

Review Video: Test Anxiety
Visit mometrix.com/academy and enter code: 100340

Important Qualification

Not all anxiety is created equal. If your test anxiety is causing major issues in your life beyond the classroom or testing center, or if you are experiencing troubling physical symptoms related to your anxiety, it may be a sign of a serious physiological or psychological condition. If this sounds like your situation, we strongly encourage you to seek professional help.

Online Resources

Due to our efforts to try to keep this book to a manageable length, we've created a link that will give you access to all of your online resources:

mometrix.com/resources719/fpgee

It's Your Moment, Let's Celebrate It!

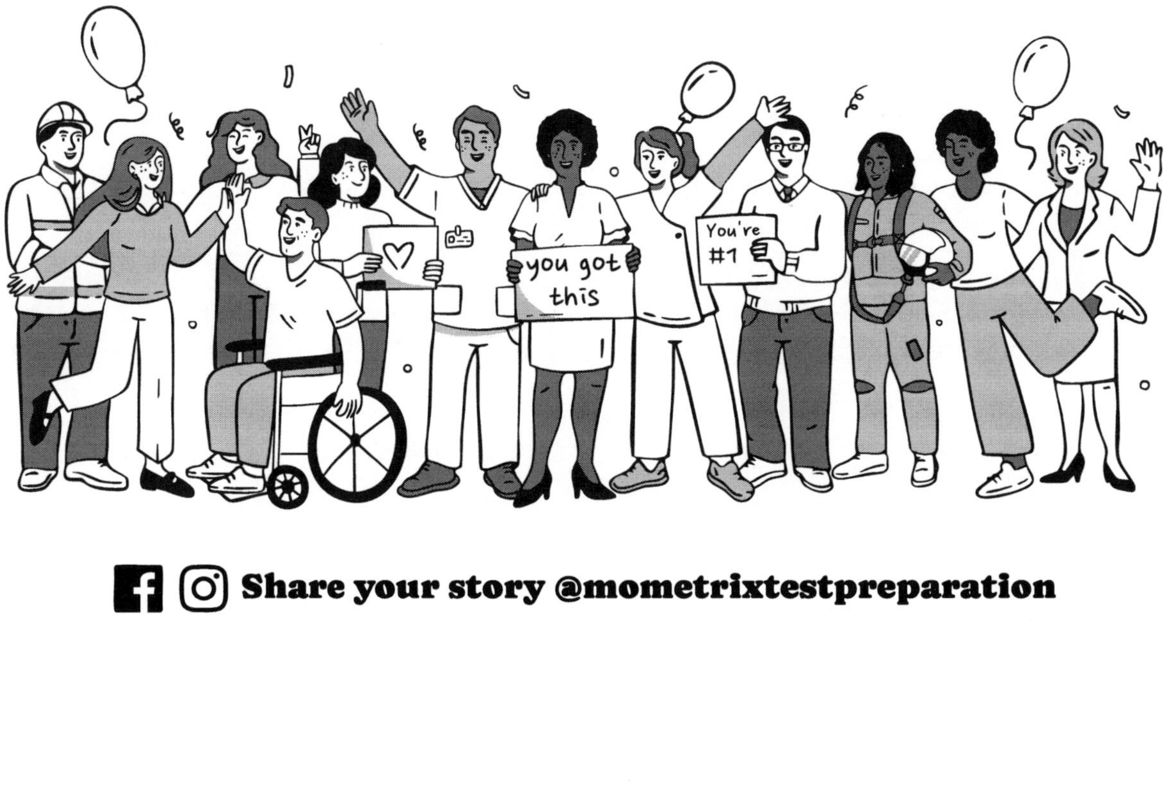

Share your story @mometrixtestpreparation